Jimmy

JIM SAYRE

PAGE PUBLISHING
Conneaut Lake, PA

First originally published by Page Publishing 2023

ISBN 979-8-88793-256-9 (pbk)
ISBN 979-8-88793-259-0 (digital)

Printed in the United States of America

Foreword

Jimmy Sayre and I were born in 1939 at Good Samaritan Hospital in Zanesville, Ohio. The hospital is no longer there, kind of like the Zanesville we grew up in.

It's a pleasure for me to write this because Jimmy is my hero. The example of his life and wise counsel and teachings have helped thousands of blind folks hope for and build better lives.

We had many adventures together coming of age in Zanesville. It was an education of learning by doing. Imagine blind little Jimmy Sayre riding a bicycle up and down the alleys of town—just amazing! And I was right there with him.

Jimmy lived across the street from the hospital, and I lived a block or so away. I can't remember when I met Jimmy for the first time, but I do remember going to nursery school with him. And then we attended kindergarten together at Westview School.

We passed from there to first grade at Lincoln Elementary. But Jimmy was losing his sight by then, so he soon after transferred to the local sight-saving school for children with vision problems. The following year, Jimmy was sent to the Ohio School for the Blind in Columbus.

We both had our disabilities. Jimmy's was more obvious. I had what would now be termed a "learning disability." Specifically, I fell far behind my peers in learning how to read and write.

We both felt we could do more than was expected of us. Yes, Jimmy was blind, but he did tons of things that folks back then didn't think blind people could do. And I was trying to prove I wasn't as dumb as many people thought. We felt that we had to do things that other kids our age couldn't or wouldn't do. You'll read about some of those escapades in Jimmy's story.

With Jimmy in Columbus at the blind school, I had my own struggles at Lincoln. By third grade there, teachers and administrators had classified me as a slow learner—my classmates just called me dumb—and insisted I repeat the grade.

However, they gave me an out. Zanesville was still largely segregated in 1947, and Lincoln was an all-white school with students from middle- to upper-class families. But there was an integrated grade school, McIntyre Elementary, not too far away, for blacks and poor whites. I was told that I could graduate to the fourth grade if I agreed to transfer there. For me, that was a no-brainier. I attended McIntyre for the fourth, fifth, and sixth grades.

When Jimmy returned to Zanesville for good to attend Roosevelt Junior High, we continued our shenanigans on a more regular basis. Occasionally that involved joy riding in "borrowed" cars. That went on until I got busted. Thank goodness Jimmy wasn't with me that night.

When you read Jimmy's story, remember the time we grew up in. The world of expectations for disabled kids was narrower back then. After all, the future for blind boys back in the 1940s was to live with a family member and maybe sell pencils and chewing gum on a street corner. And for dumb me, there was always life as a ditchdigger.

But Jimmy broke past society's expectations by getting a master's degree. He worked with rehab programs for Services for the Blind in Wisconsin and Ohio, through the years improving the lives of thousands of folks with impaired vision and becoming a living model for blind people.

And he has always been a great ambassador to the sighted, to help them better understand blind folks' needs and ambitions.

Those two achievements are themes that run through the length of Jimmy Sayre's remarkable story.

In his story, you'll read about Jimmy's struggles in college. I had my own, of course, and I also did what I had to do to graduate. Later, I became a navy SEAL officer, and after serving eleven years in the navy, I pioneered the use of the electronic funds transfer service. Upon retirement at age 64, I built a small resort, Casamar Suites, which I still manage in Puerto Escondido, Oaxaca, Mexico.

Because of our disabilities—in spite of them, who can say?—Jimmy and I became close friends and pals, and we have continued this relationship all our lives. I wrote this foreword on Jimmy's dining room table at his home on Wilmer Street in Zanesville.

I complimented Jimmy for sharing his life story so far, and he assured me the statute of limitation has expired on our childhood adventures.

For sure, the world for blind folks is better because of Jimmy's work and his many contributions. I know you will enjoy reading about his life's adventures and accomplishments.

What blessings!

—Willits Sawyer
Zanesville, Ohio
September 2019

Preface

In 1803, so they say, in the Muskingum Valley an infant town lay,
Like an unpolished diamond, concealing its worth,
Was Zanesville, Ohio, my heaven on earth.

Oh, the river gave power to drive the grist mill
From its bowels came fine clay for the potters' craft wheel,
The title Clay City was given in mirth
To Zanesville, Ohio, my heaven on earth

The years rolled along then, as they always do
The steamboats came west and the railroads did too
The town grew important, expanded its girth
Oh, Zanesville, Ohio, my heaven on earth

If like me you were born there, like me you were raised,
If like me you've traveled, then like me you've been amazed
To find yourself longing for your land of birth
Oh, Zanesville, Ohio, my heaven on earth

I wrote that song some fifty years ago, when I was living and working in Wisconsin and feeling homesick. Being homesick for Zanesville has been a regular refrain in my life whenever I've been away.

Zanesville lies in east central Ohio, some fifty miles east of Columbus out I-70. It had about forty thousand residents when I grew up there in the 1940s and '50s. It's a town of history, an early settlement in the Northwest Territory and briefly capital of Ohio in the early nineteenth century.

It's a town of great significance to me and my story. I was born there in 1939, the last of three sons in a family with long roots in Muskingum and Guernsey counties.

Zanesville is important to me because the town as a whole and its people accepted me, supported me, and even reveled in my successes as a totally blind individual.

I'm telling my story because of the many requests I've had to do so through the years from friends, professionals with whom I've worked, and even casual acquaintances. They felt that the things I've accomplished—whether socially, scholastically, or professionally—were doubly surprising, some even say uncanny, because I did those things as a blind person.

Chapter 1: The Early Years

Some of my earliest recollections were of me and my mother leaving Zanesville, going off to see different eye doctors in different cities across the country in the hope that they would be able to do something to save what little vision I had. We were always glad to get back home.

Back in 1939, the practice at birth was, if a doctor wasn't present, to have the mother hold back the child—to delay birth—-until the doctor arrived. Speculation is that the pressure on my head, being held back for about half an hour before the doctor arrived, damaged the interior workings of my ocular system, resulting in gradual but total blindness at the age of six.

At that time, the World War II years, blindness was due mainly to birth defects and accidents. There were fewer blind adults because people didn't live as long as we do now. Most blindness occurs later in life, caused by different diseases, with diabetes the number 1 cause of blindness in the United States. Macular degeneration occurs later in life too. People are living longer, so they're having more of the age-related causes of blindness.

As it became clear that my eyesight would deteriorate, eventually ending in blindness, my family—mother, father, and two older brothers—was devastated. But they were equally determined that I would lead a life full of love, acceptance, and help wherever necessary so that I could lead a normal life—with one notable exception.

I don't mean that they sat down and devised a program to follow—we must do this, we must do that—but my mother, especially, possessed an unusual amount of common sense. My brother Bob was uncommonly sensitive too. He spent many hours with me, even though he wasn't around much, being sixteen years older. Bob was graduating from high school when I was still an infant, and soon after he was off to Europe and service in World War II.

Mom received a letter from Bob when he was somewhere in Europe during WWII after she had told him that I would soon be totally blind and that the doctor had told her there was nothing that could be done medically to prevent it.

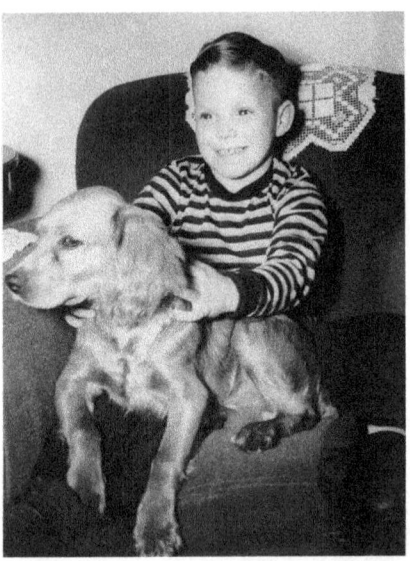

A young Jimmy with his cocker spaniel, Tawny.

The letter from Bob expressed his concern and dismay over the news, of course, but he declared in that letter that he would take care of me no matter what. That always stuck in my mind. Bob was sixteen years older than me and was really more of a father figure than my own dad ever was.

I remember Bob and especially my mother reading stories to me, reading books beyond my years, playing ball, doing other activities. One vivid memory involves Bob spending many hours trying to teach me how to tie my shoes. I recall being frustrated to the point of tears, but he insisted, cajoled, encouraged, and finally succeeded in teaching me how to accomplish the rite of passage common to all small children—being able to tie one's shoes.

In the neighborhood around my home, there were many other children about my age, and even though my vision at that time was severely limited, they learned to accept me for what I was. If they saw me run into a tree or misjudge a turn into a sidewalk and run into a bush, they accepted it, maybe laughed a little like I did, and we all went on.

We lived a more or less normal life in the neighborhood as children. We played games like kick the can, hide-and-seek, cops and robbers, cowboys and Indians, red rover—the whole gamut. And I was right in there with them, doing what I could to participate, which usually was almost completely.

I remember when I was four or five, we'd go to a filling station near the house to buy soda and potato chips. The people who worked there learned that I could find the door and come in. They'd help me find what I was looking for and apparently not think much of it once they were used to seeing me.

One day I was sitting on a corner near the station, at two of the busier streets of the neighborhood, listening and watching the traffic go by, what I could still see at the time. There was a lady waiting for the city bus standing there, and she started to talk to me. She asked me who I was, and I told her I was Jimmy Sayre. The next day in the local newspaper, in a column called The Old Gossip, there was an account of our meeting.

Apparently the woman I spoke to was the writer of the column. The story ran with a picture of me in my bib overalls and striped shirt, resembling the current-day Dennis the Menace, captioned "Little Jimmy Sayre, sitting on the corner of Maple and Adair." That was my first claim to fame in the newspaper, as far as I know.

I always had a good memory and a sharp mind. In fact, members of the family would ask me when they were trying to remember something, and nine out of ten times I could remember what they were trying to. One of my earliest memories was my mother teaching me a recipe by memory, how to make fudge. I presented that while standing on a chair so people could see me at one of her circle meetings.

Of course, when I was a kid, I had to remember everything in my head. There were no handheld tape recorders at the time, and of course, it would be half a century until computers and tablets came around. In fact, it wasn't until I went to the Ohio State School for the Blind in Columbus that I was introduced to the first technology blind people could use to make notes: a slate and stylus that allowed us to write braille by hand on small punch cards. But first you had to learn braille, not an easy chore. More on the blind school to come.

In addition, I was always musical and could sing at a very early age. In fact, my mother had me entertaining places when I was two and a half to three years old. I could remember the words and carry a tune, and I guess I was cute, so it made a nice package. I went on to develop my musical talent more fully later in life.

As I said earlier, some of my earliest memories were of me and my mother traveling to other cities in Ohio and West Virginia, even Johns Hopkins in Baltimore, Maryland, one time to see if there were doctors around who could help save my vision, whatever I had left, or heal the problem. Unfortunately, there was no help to be found.

I remember the last doctor we saw, a doctor in Columbus. I'll never forget what he said. He told my mother that he hated to say it, but it was his opinion that I would go totally blind and that there was nothing that could be done to prevent it. He went on to say that she should enroll me at the State School for the Blind in Columbus.

At this point in my young life, I had gone to nursery school and kindergarten program in Zanesville public schools. I had become adjusted to the situation and was able to compensate, for the most part, and do most of the tasks asked of me.

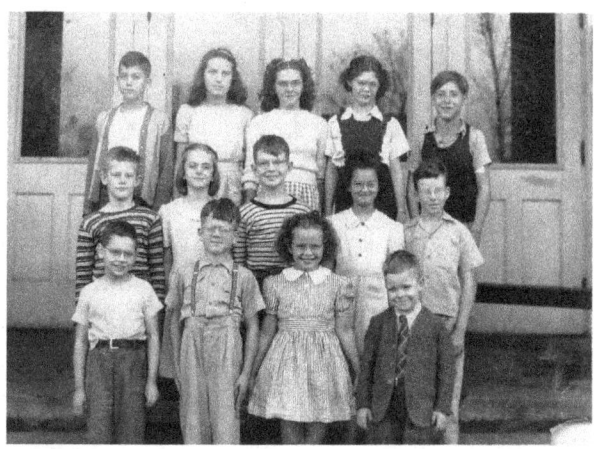

Jimmy's sight saving school, which included children from several grades. Jim is the youngest, front row right, with tie and jacket.

But by the time first grade rolled around, I couldn't see well enough to do the assignments.

So I was referred to the "sight-saving" school in Zanesville, where they used large-print books and large maps to attempt to educate kids with limited vision. At that point, though, I was unable to see well enough to accomplish the sight-saving assignments either.

I remember coming home from sight-saving classes one afternoon around Christmastime, I guess I was six, and asking my mom, "Hey, turn on the light."

My mom said, "The light is on, Jimmy."

During that day, while I was at school, I lost whatever little vision I had left. From that day on, I would be totally blind.

One of my first memorable friends was Willits, who attended nursery school and kindergarten at the same time I did. He lived about a block and a half away, and we were readily accessible to each other. We did a lot of things together at that age and all through life—we're still friends today. Willits went on to become one of the first navy SEALs, then called frogmen.

Another friend, a pal I made in sight-saving class, was Guy. We became fast friends and did a lot of things together. Guy was from a rather poor family, didn't have much money. My mother, who wanted us to experience normalcy in life, would give us money, pay Guy's way to go to the movies, for instance, on Saturday. We'd go to the movies. Of course I could listen and more or less know what was going on. He and I would walk downtown, about a mile or so, or ride the bus.

One of my excursions with Guy became my first experience at shoplifting. As I said, Guy was from what was referred to in those days as a poor family. I stayed overnight once, and Guy and I went out to the local market. Guy stole some candy, which I readily helped consume. I wasn't sure at that time where it came from. I had my suspicions, but since he got away with it, well, it was okay with me.

We would go swimming during the summer at the local pool where all the other kids our age went. I took swimming lessons there, too, and was given verbal directions when the instructor was teaching strokes, visually, to the other swimmers. I learned to swim, anyway, and have never drowned, so I must have been effective.

There was a skating rink in town where a lot of kids would go on Saturdays. Guy and I went there, and I learned how to roll-er-skate. I had several wrecks with other people, but they seemed to learn how to watch out for me and avoid me. It was a fairly good experience all in all.

Learning how to skate helped develop my sense of balance, which often is affected when one loses vision, something I learned at a later date.

As said earlier, the kids in the neighborhood would play a lot of games, and I would, of course, participate. I knew the neighborhood really well and was able to run and knew good places to hide. One time, I remember, we were playing kick the can. I left my hiding place and came running in to jump over the can and free everyone who'd been caught up to that point. Well, I thought I knew where the can was, but it wasn't where I thought it was. I bet I was a real spectacle jumping over a can that wasn't there!

Another day we put on a "circus" in the yard behind the alley where a friend of mine named Brad lived. We invited all the family members to come, the mothers of the different participants. We had wagon races, and I was the "motor," pushing the wagon rather than guiding it. I didn't care because I was involved. Another of my jobs in the circus was to be the high-flying man. I got in the swing, kicked myself as high as possible, and then jumped out. I was daring enough to do it even if I couldn't see how far down it was. I didn't break anything, so I count it as a success.

I was always stronger than the other kids, strong for my age. I used to shinny up the support poles of the swing set and sit on top of it. Not many of the other kids could do that, so I felt like I was really king of the neighborhood at that point, being able to do what the others couldn't. Of course, we would have foot races in the alley behind our house that bisected the block. We'd have races, jumping contests, all that type of thing, and I was always pretty good at that, and pretty fast. As long as I was on the gravel bed of the alley, I was able to know more or less where I was and able to compete, usually successfully.

I said earlier that I was always a ham and would show off whenever I could, singing and performing by reciting recipes and other memory-related activities. In the years before TV, radio, of course, was very important in Americans' lives. There was a radio talent show, the *Horrace Heidt Show*, where people from all over the country would compete, and the best of them would, hopefully, go on to stardom in the entertainment field.

The show came to Zanesville one year, and I was invited by the junior Chamber of Commerce, the sponsor of the event, to be on stage and be part of the welcome committee, which consisted of dignitaries from the city, walking on stage with Horrace Heidt and welcoming him. People in the city administration asked me to take part, and my mom and I got to sit behind the stage and meet a lot of the stars traveling in the troupe with Heidt including some rather well-known names in show business. Dick Contino, who was known nationally as a virtuoso on the accordion, and a midget named Johnny who was featured in an ad for Philip Morris cigarettes, they were backstage too. They befriended me, giving me signed autographed pictures, which I still must have somewhere. I can't really enjoy the pictures, but I did enjoy meeting them and being with them backstage.

Earlier I mentioned my brother Bob working with me to tie my shoes and other tasks dealing with grooming and dressing. He also worked with me on directions, on following sounds. One time he bought a bow-and-arrow kit for kids, one with suction cups on the end so that no one could get hurt. We'd get out in the backyard, and Bob would stand up by the side of the house and pound away on it so that I could hear where he was and shoot toward the noise. Of course, if I hit him, it wouldn't hurt too much with the suction cups. It certainly helped me formulate my body's relationship with sound direction and how you could throw at a sound or shoot at a sound and hit it.

Bob and Mom and sometimes my other brother, Ken, would bounce a ball on the sidewalk in the backyard, and I would work at it to the point where I could hit a ball on the up-bounce with a bat. That was my own semblance of baseball.

Later when I was a counselor at YMCA camp, I was able to pitch softball by having the batter speak, and I was able to be very accurate in getting him a pitch to hit. That amazed a lot of people, and of course it made the papers: "A Blind Man Pitches Softball—Successfully!"

As I mentioned before, we had a lot of kids near our ages in the neighborhood, and we would play from dawn to dusk like kids have for millennia. One day a girl that lived next door, Gretchen, decided that she was going to teach me how to ride a bicycle. We borrowed the bike of a playmate, and she walked with me up and down the sidewalk, teaching me how to balance the bike.

After a bit, I got the hang of it. And that led to a feat that astonished the other kids: eventually I learned how to ride a bike up the sidewalk and turn into our front walk between two sticker bushes without hitting either bush. Other kids—fully sighted kids— were usually unable to match me and ended up in the sticker bushes. I accomplished my little magic trick using what I would later call "echolocation."

I knew that if I was riding up from the south, right before the turn into the sidewalk, there was a large tree. The sound of the bicycle and the movement of my body echoed off that tree, and then I knew I had to make a split-second turn into the sidewalk. I got to the point that I could do it successfully nine out of ten times. I knew it was due to the echolocation from the tree because if I rode toward the house from the other direction, from the north, there was no tree to orient me. When I wanted to impress people, I always made sure to ride up from the south. People really thought I was slick!

I had figured out at an even earlier age that when I moved, my body created sounds. Sounds, when they bounce off solid objects, create echoes. At some point, I noticed that I could use these echoes to sense objects in front of me, walls or buildings, for example. In crossing a street, I figured out that the sounds of my footsteps would bounce back off the curb and help me sense what was around me and where I was in the street. One day, as a tyke holding my mother's hand to cross the street, I raised my little foot to step onto the curb, and Mom asked me, "How did you know to do that?" That's echolocation.

It's a very simple process. The navy uses it as sonar, bats use it as their own travel instruments, and I, over the years, developed it to a very high degree. In fact, I owe a lot of my mobility skills, as all blind people do, to echolocation. I just happened to develop it to a little higher degree, a higher sensitivity than most blind people who use other means of travel identification, such as guide dogs or canes.

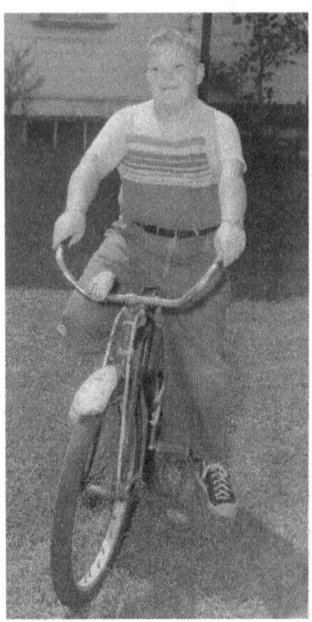

Pre-teen Jimmy riding his bicycle around the neighborhood.

I was able, as a kid, to ride a bicycle for several years around my end of Zanesville, mainly using sidewalks and alleys. The alleys in town became my private bike trails. Most of the alleys had gravel surfaces, and I could tell whenever I got off the gravel to get the bike back on the cinders and keep going.

Later on, I learned that if I wore hard heels or heel plates on my shoes that those aids would create a more distinct echo. I developed this skill to the point where I could detect a two-inch bump in the sidewalk, telephone poles, trees—any solid object of any size. I also had very good balance and for some reason, always had an excellent sense of direction. All these skills allowed me to travel independently through my years in school, later in college, and even later in my professional life.

As I got older and my education increased, I learned that academics gave professional terms to the skills I'd been developing as a youngster: orientation and mobility, skills that are certainly important parts of becoming adjusted to being blind or seriously visually impaired. Orientation, in short, is the title given to becoming familiar with your living arrangement—apartment, bedroom, house, office, gymnasium—anywhere you spend regular, substantial amounts of time in.

Just like any other phase of life, there are those who are good at orientation and those who, for whatever reason, have problems. Some people, and I would include myself, orient to a new situation very quickly. Then there are others who never become familiar with their surrounding and continue to have difficulties getting around. And, too, some blind people have medical problems, such as traumatic brain injuries, that limit their ability to develop more fully these orientation skills.

Mobility, the other half of the equation, is the art of learning how to travel independently, either by walking, using public transportation, or developing a network of friends and family to arrange transportation from one point to another. About the only way to progress in orientation is through repetition and allowing the visually impaired person to familiarize himself with his own environment.

Since it is impossible to use vision as your basic sense in achieving mobility, a blind person learns to use aids and other senses to bolster your lack of vision. These include hearing, obviously, and our tactile sense—feeling things—along with an acute memory and awareness of landmarks in our environment. These can be the whir of fans, bumps and gaps in sidewalks, and regular smells.

I've always been able to be 95 percent independent in getting from place to place and doing what I had to do, especially after being accompanied the first time in a new place by a sighted person. If no one was available, I'd use public transportation or ask other friends for a ride.

As I said, I was able to pitch softball at the local YMCA camp where I went in summers as a camper and later worked as a counselor and camp director. The umpire would stand with me on the mound rather than at the plate. He'd catch the ball when the catcher threw it back for the next pitch, then hand it to me. I'd ask the batter to speak, and once he did, I'd throw the next pitch. It was fun, and everybody enjoyed it, especially me, and they thought I was pretty cool.

I mentioned earlier that my long life has been fun a lot of the time and full of funny incidents. One of them happened when I was seven or eight years old. It included a large boxer dog named Super, belonging to a neighbor who didn't seem to have much interest in its whereabouts or conduct. Super was often seen knocking down neighborhood kids, not because he was malicious but because he was so big and enthusiastic.

One day Willits manipulated his private parts until Super appeared to have a seizure. We didn't exactly know what happened, but from that day on Super was highly interested in Willits and seemed to be one of his fast friends.

Another incident with Willits involved his cat, Charlie Chaplin, so called because he had a little mustache like the movie star. We wanted to know if cats always landed on their feet, so he decided to launch Charlie from a second-story window to test this hypothesis. Unfortunately for Charlie, he didn't land on his feet but quickly jumped up and ran away from the scene. Needless to say, he gave Willits a wide berth after that.

I mentioned attending nursery school with Willits, held in the basement of a home about five blocks from my own. He and I would walk together to the school, which lasted about three hours a day, and enter through a separate door to the basement. The lady that owned the house where the nursery school met was a friend of my mother's. One day I told Willits that it would be funny if we snuck upstairs and hid, then scared the lady of the house when she got home.

It was taboo for the kids to go the upstairs part of the house, but for some odd reason, the basement door wasn't locked. We snuck upstairs and hid in the closet. When the lady came home, we jumped out and shouted, "Boo!" Of course, we later caught holy hell for scaring the lady and for being upstairs, where we weren't allowed. My mom found out about it, obviously, and I was duly punished. I think I had to sit on a chair or something for five minutes.

I was pretty inquisitive as a child and, I thought, pretty smart. We had a pantry in the kitchen where all the cans and pans and other items were stored. One day I decided to climb the shelves, using the shelves as a ladder. Finally, after a few attempts, I reached the top shelf, where I found a square box, which I opened to find candy! I proceeded to devour the contents, not knowing that the box contained not regular chocolate but ex-lax! Well, you can guess what happened. Mom called the doctor, who said he didn't think it would hurt me.

"But you'll be busy for the next two or three days," he told her. From all accounts, she was.

Family Motivation

People have asked me from time to time where I got my motivation to push ahead, to do things that seemed beyond the reach of a blind person. I've thought a lot about that during the years. As in the case with most people, I think, my motivation came from the desire to please one family member—that would be Mom—and to prove another wrong, that being my dad, Leo, as I refer to him.

Mom was the type who made a big deal out of me riding a bicycle around or things like that. She loved that: "Oh, that's wonderful," "you're amazing," and so on. That was sweet music to my ears.

Mom never told me not to do something. She would never say, "You can't do this." She might say, "You could get hurt," or "Jimmy, be careful!" like any mother would, but she never dissuaded me from doing something. That was great, because I always had the urge to do things, and I had at least her unspoken approval to go for it.

And she was ahead of her time in seeing that blind people needed to be integrated into the sighted world. I was the only kid in the blind school at that time who was from out of town—whose family didn't live in Columbus—who went home every weekend. Most of the kids were there from the end of summer to Christmas and then from New Year's to Easter, Easter to the start of summer.

That situation, unfortunately, led to them being institutionalized. When you learn to live in and become used to living in a blind-only institution instead of your home, your community, it diminishes your ability to live in a sighted world. Everything was designed to make it easier for us to function. You get accustomed to living in the world of the visually impaired. But that's not how the world outside functions. And my mom knew that instinctively.

From Leo, however, I got negative incentive. He always made me feel that I was inferior, that he was embarrassed by having a child who was less than perfect.

My brother Kenny, five years older, was always a really good athlete, and Leo poured all kinds of praise and acclamation over him. I never got any of that, just cold silence a lot of the time. About my bike-riding exploits or my mentions in the newspaper, Leo never said shit. And he was quick to give me hell if I knocked over a glass of water or something. You'd think he caught me robbing a bank. Even later, when I went to study for my master's degree, which no one in my family had ever done, I overheard him tell one person that he didn't know what in the hell I was doing, that I was down in Tennessee wasting my time. But when I got the degree and a good job, he had to eat his words.

Leo's negativity just made me more determined to succeed, to do what I wanted to do the way I wanted to do it. I remember telling my nephew one time as he lamented the strain of stubbornness that runs through Sayre men, "Stubborn! Hell, that's one of our best traits!"

As I said, I had several articles about me in the local Zanesville papers—believe it or not, there were three papers in Zanesville when I was a kid: the morning *Signal*, the afternoon *Times-Recorder*, and the *News*—about me going to Camp Moores, pitching softball, swimming, that kind of thing. Once they came out and did a picture study of me, following me around on a typical day taking pictures. It became a picture feature in the papers.

I also got a Bulova Braille watch from an ABC network show called *Kid and Company*. They found out about me when a neighbor who was editor of the *Zanesville News* sent my story to them; I never had any direct contact with anyone on the show. I remember watching it: they showed pictures of me riding a bike, playing sandlot football, pitching softball, and the like. I remember some kids at the Y telling me that they saw it, too. Pretty cool to be on national TV when there were only three channels.

Chapter 2: The Ohio School for the Blind

Earlier I said that I recalled hearing the last ophthalmologist I saw in Columbus telling my mom that I would soon be totally blind and that she should enroll me at the Ohio State School for the Blind. When I was seven, she did.

That started a cycle in my life that was riddled with a lot of really bad homesickness. I was uprooted from my family and my neighborhood and sent to this residential school sixty miles or so away, where I was to live and receive my schooling. I'd learn to use braille books, which allowed us visually impaired, sightless kids to learn our ABC's, so to speak. After lengthy training in braille, we could use it as the sighted world uses print.

As I said, this was a very painful and uprooting part of my life, having to leave home when I was just seven years old and being thrown screaming and kicking into a brand-new—and often cruel and frightening—situation. Blind children enrolled in the school would go there and live during the school year in a dormitory setting, which for most of us was an uprooting and very traumatic experience.

I really never realized how strong homesickness could be. Often I found myself crying at the most inopportune time during the day, especially when I wasn't busy doing something in school. I would go to my dormitory room and sit on my chair next to my bed with my face buried in the pillow and cry. I didn't realize why I had been uprooted from my family and sent to this place where I was some-what bullied by others.

At one point, I thought I had a foolproof scheme to bankrupt the blind school and get returned to my Zanesville home. My seven-year-old mind came up with the idea that turning the lights on and off, which my brother Kenny and I had been told many times by our parents was a waste of money, would cause the school to go bankrupt. Then I would be sent home, where I belonged. Alas, I sat for hours in my dormitory room flicking the switch on and off, but no financial collapse occurred. There at the blind school I stayed.

I remember one situation where we were playing, and all at once I had the most painful experience in my life. One of the bullies had slapped me across the face with the rubber tread from a toy tank for no reason at all that I could discern. I don't think I'd ever had anything hurt more at that time. It wasn't only painful, it was very frightening, coming from a comfortable, secure home as I did.

Another time, one of the older boys thought I hadn't been initiated into the dormitory life as much as I should have been. He decided to take it upon himself to kick my ass. I understood that this was going to happen, so I hid in my dorm room under my bed in hopes that he wouldn't find me. Well, he had a person with him who had some vision who helped him find me. That kid told the older bully to get under the bed with me, where he proceeded to whale on me with his fists.

I screamed as loud as I could for the dormitory matron, the lady in charge of us on the floor. She came to my rescue after I had only been hit two or three times. I soon learned that the only way to avoid being beat up was to be able to fight back, to give as good as you received or better. Soon I became a fairly effective fighter for my own preservation.

The dorms were set up in different sections: younger kids, which I was, say ages 5 through 10; medium age, which was 10 to 14; and high schoolers, who were upstairs and supervised by other matrons.

The rooms had five beds in each room, five lockers, one for each student, five chairs, one table. Needless to say, it was a very close living arrangement. We showered three or four times a week, not every day. We were marched to and from meals by our matrons, and in some ways it was very similar to being in prison.

As I said before, and I can't really emphasize this too much, I was completely overcome, especially in the first few years, by homesickness. But I must say that my life was much better off than most of the kids who were there almost the whole year. Their contact with a normal family life was, of course, interrupted and replaced by institutional living.

Here again my mother's common sense and her desire to have me live as normal a life as possible led her to have me return home every single weekend, rather than leave me languishing in the residential situation. So I was able to maintain a semblance of normalcy in my life and maintain contact with the sighted world and my normal home life.

One weekend, when I was nine or ten, Mom decided that I should go to the YMCA downtown on Saturdays, when they had programs for kids. She rode the bus with me downtown the first couple of times, and then I asked her to let me do it by myself.

So that first time I left home, walked to the corner where the bus stopped, and got on. The bus drivers knew me from trips with Mom, and they didn't think anything was amiss. I got on the bus and told them I wanted off at Fifth and Main and asked them to tell me when we got there. I got off and walked down to the corner at Fifth Street. I could tell when I got to the corner because I heard the echo from a building there, so I knew to turn left down Fifth, and right before I got to the Y, there was an alley. I crossed the alley, heard the echoes from the Y building, and went to the second set of wide steps. I went up the steps and into the building.

There's a funny story in that, and I didn't find out about it until many years later. That first time I went to the Y by myself, Mom followed me without me knowing it. She shushed the bus driver when she got on, and he played along. But once she saw I could do it, it was cool. She allowed me to do it by myself.

She was a mother and wanted her boy home as much as possible. She would cry as hard as I did every Monday morning when I got on the bus to go back to Columbus and Friday night became the joyful night of the week because I was coming home.

Those bus drivers on the Columbus-to-Zanesville route became important people in my life. Since the same drivers made the trip back and forth from Columbus—that's every weekend when school was in session from first grade through seventh grade—they all got to know me, and I knew them all by their first names. They looked out for me to the point where they began buying things for me for Christmas. When I was in the fifth grade, they pooled their money and bought me my first clarinet. Mom called a reporter she knew who came by to write a story. And they bought me my first braille watch, too. They worked for the Lake Shore bus system; it's not in business anymore.

The Lake Shore drivers also sponsored a newspaper vending machine at the Zanesville station with my picture and a sign saying "Proceeds go to provide gifts for Jim Sayre." They used that to raise money to buy me Christmas presents. You bought a paper, and some of the money went to them to pay for my gifts. They did a hell of a job for me.

To get home on Fridays, the blind school would call me a cab that took me to the bus station in downtown Columbus. Once I got there, a redcap, a porter, would find a seat for me and then put me on the right bus when it was time. And of course, when I got to Zanesville, I knew Mom would be there to meet me.

It was a local bus, no Interstate 70 in those days. It stopped in every little town on Route 40: Reynoldsburg, Kirkersville, Hebron, Jacktown, Brownsville, Gratiot, then finally Zanesville. From there it went on to Cambridge and Wheeling and towns in between.

I rode that Lake Shore bus to Zanesville from Columbus on Friday nights, making the return trip on Monday morning and staying at the school from then until Friday. This arrangement, of course, led to sorrow on Monday morning and joy on Friday night. I really looked forward to my weekends at home and wouldn't have missed them for the world.

I think my ability to maintain regular contact with the sighted world, thanks to those weekend trips home, helped me to adjust to living in the sighted world as a blind person later in life. All that helped me to become, later in life, a good student in college and a productive person in the workaday world. I learned how to compensate for my impairment in getting along with sighted people with the senses I had left, especially my hearing, so that they wouldn't think I was a freak.

In that manner, I was accepted by sighted people and allowed—even encouraged—to try things usually not done by a visually impaired person. At the downtown YMCA on Saturday mornings, I played with sighted kids in the gym, on the track, and in the swimming pool. Later on we socialized together, just having common conversations, watching movies, even trying to play Ping-Pong and pool. I boxed and wrestled with the sighted kids, played dodgeball, and more. And I was able to participate in all these games with them. I also ran as part of relay teams on the track that hung about thirty feet above the gym floor. The track had a low guard rail, so one of the Y assistants would run with me so that I wouldn't fall over it while I made my way around.

Don't get me wrong, looking back I'm glad my parents made me go to the blind school even though it was emotionally painful and traumatic in a lot of ways. Regimentation was a part of life there, and I could have been another institutionalized kid, too. Lucky for me, I had a mother determined to keep me in her life and part of the sighted world in Zanesville.

As I said, at the blind school, we were supervised by house matrons, but one person cannot adequately supervise thirty or forty children twenty-four hours a day. Of course, six or seven hours of each weekday we were in class, but that left a lot of time for us to develop habits, some of which were not good. There was arguing, fighting, and other types of treachery. We did establish good friendships, but there was always the underlying threat of violence and bully rule.

One of the most important things that happened to me at the blind school was the exposure and training I got in music there. I seemed to have a strong talent for music at an early age, and it was encouraged and developed, in part, at the school.

I took piano lessons for years, but I didn't really enjoy it, didn't really catch on to it very well. Finally, I gave that up. However, I was introduced to the clarinet and became proficient playing it, along with related woodwinds like the tenor and alto saxophones. I was in the school band at the blind school and later in orchestras at public schools.

I was blessed with a good singing voice from an early age. My mom used to tell me that I had been singing in public since I was two and a half years old! I guess she noticed that I could sing at any early age and showed me off to people in the area by having me sing at social events and organizations she was involved with.

I was in the chorus at the school for the blind and later in vocal groups in the Zanesville public school system.

Music was, has been, and always will be a very important part of my life. My initial exposure to music at the blind school led to it being part of my life as I grew up and joined professional bands for the next half century. Dance bands, dance combos, choral groups and more—I loved it all. Music not only let me participate in an activity that I love, it helped me earn extra money.

Later in life, mainly when I was living in Wisconsin, I composed several songs, most of which dealt with Zanesville, where I grew up. I wrote the song that I quoted in the preface from my time in Wisconsin and included it in a record album I made.

It's not true that blind people are automatically good at music, that the time we spend relying on and improving our hearing to navigate in the world produces good musicians. There are blind people who can't sing or play an instrument.

But in some phases of music—improvisation, for instance—I think blindness to a degree helps. We can't read music, obviously, so learning pieces relies entirely on memory. At the blind school, the director of the band would get us together in groups—like all the clarinets—and drill us on our parts, to memorize them. We had band concerts where people would come from all over the state to hear us. We were great!

Others have said, and it's true, that being in the band in a state blind school was like being on the football team in sighted schools. It's true, it was a big deal and a big source of personal confidence and pride to band members.

The year after I left, the blind school actually added a competitive sport to activities for boys there—wrestling. And they really got into it. There were state tournaments, like the Wisconsin blind school would come wrestle us in Ohio. And they'd wrestle sighted schools, too. The only difference is that in the beginning of the match, the wrestlers don't approach each other, they begin in the position where the wrestlers touch each other with one on his hands and knees and the other one squatting above him.

I also learned at the blind school that I enjoyed learning. I had a quick mind and usually caught on to new concepts without too much trouble. In fact, I found education so easy that I'm afraid I coasted through a lot of classes, achieving enough to get by but, I'm sure, not doing as well as I could have.

Learning Braille

I know that many sighted friends who are mystified by blind people's ability to "read" braille with their fingertips, since the concept is so foreign, and apparently inconceivable, to them. First of all, let me explain that braille has no relationship whatsoever with print, cursive, or any other written symbols. Braille are symbols in themselves, formulated to be read tactilely, by touching the raised dots, in braille form only.

I entered the blind school in the first grade, which was when young blind students were first introduced to braille, using what were called at that time as pegboards. Keep in mind that the most important aspect of learning braille and being able to use it well demands that you develop the ability to feel the differences in the raised dots with the tips of your fingers.

A braille cell generates six dots—three dots down in two vertical rows. The braille alphabet and numbering system is formulated by different configurations of those six dots. Example: the letter A is one dot at the top left of the cell. That particular dot is known as dot 1. The rest of the letters of the alphabet are denoted by different configurations of those six dots.

Numbers are designated by using a number sign in combination with braille signs *A* through *J* as the numbers 1 through 10. For instance, the letter *A*—the dot at the top left of the braille cell—

becomes the number 1 when you put a number sign in front of it. *B* with a number sign in front becomes a 2 and so on, until you get to the letter *J*, which is 0. In this way, braille accounts for the ten single numbers that are used to make all numbers.

Other configurations of the dots are also used to indicate punctuation.

Anyway, the pegboards that we learned braille on were rectangular wooden boards about a half inch thick, about six by ten inches. The boards had braille cells drilled into them, into which a student would place round-headed brass tacks to formulate the dots.

The beginning braille student—remember we were in first grade—starts learning to read by touch using very large dots. Over time the size of the dots is decreased until you are able to read standard dot size.

Then, as students progressed into higher grades, they are eventually introduced to contracted braille—braille "shorthand." They've taken in the most used combinations in English, *–ance* or *–ence*, for instance, and made shortcuts to cover that sequence of letters. Or a word even. Like *father* is dot-5 F, and *mother* is dot-5 M. Quicker than spelling out the whole word.

To further complicate matters, to reproduce braille, especially back in my day, to reproduce it for our own use, mostly for making short notes, we used a slate and stylus. The slate is about the size of cell phone, into which a fitted piece of paper is inserted. To make braille notes, you use the stylus, which has a sharp tip, to punch the paper. That action produces raised dots into the underside of the paper. That's the key point: the raised dots are made on the underside of the paper.

And that's where it gets complicated. Blind people feel braille dots from left to right. But because you need to turn the paper over to be able to feel the raised dots made by the stylus, you must poke holes into the paper from right to left, the opposite of how you'll read it.

In other words, to be able to read your notes correctly, you must conceptualize in your mind how the raised holes you make with your stylus will read once the paper is turned over!

That all sounds incredibly difficult, but you learn to do what you have to do very quickly. I still use a slate and stylus to make notes to myself, for less-used phone numbers, for example. For numbers I call frequently, I still memorize them.

Now, of course, the development and widespread distribution of assistive computer technology is changing the relationship, the usefulness, of braille to blind people.

For example, *Reader's Digest* used to be published in braille. You know the size of a *Reader's Digest*? You can stick it in your pocket. But it took four volumes about the size of a Columbus phone book to make a monthly *Reader's Digest*. Four volumes! That's how bulky it is. So it's impractical insofar as bulk, it used to be impractical in terms of production, and it's impractical in the amount of time it takes to read something.

Unfortunately, even contracted braille—braille shorthand—is still uncomfortably bulky. I don't think braille will ever be phased out, but it's impractical. There are so many better ways to do things these days.

Today my iPhone reads my mail for me. That's just one indication of how far technology has come. You open up the program, tap it twice, and it uses the camera in the phone to read your material. I put my mail in a reading stand, like a music stand, to keep the letter steady when I point the phone at it.

Being able to listen to material online through innovations in computer reading, like my iPhone app for reading mail, is making braille obsolete. The purists don't like that, but braille is becoming obsolete. I don't care what anybody says. It's happening.

For instance, a good braille reader, using shorthand braille, takes four times longer than a sighted print reader to read the same text. But it only takes me twice as long to listen to text as it would a sighted person to read the same material. So if you listen to it instead of using braille, you're saving twice as much time. Or to put it another way, by listening to a print reader you're only wasting half as much time as you would by reading braille.

The onset of computer advances, with Siri and Alexa voices and the like, is speedily making braille obsolete. The purists don't wish to hear this, but it's a fact. If you have a talking computer, you don't need braille anymore to obtain, store, and use information.

Back to the blind school. I found two courses there extremely interesting: typing and woodshop. The woodshop instructor, Mr. Petzinger, was a highly accomplished blind person and imparted much knowledge that served me throughout life, especially concerning the need for organization.

He preached through the years the importance of organization for blind people. You should have a special place for every specific thing, he said, and always keep that thing in its special place. In other words, when you're using something, a tool or an object—anything—put it back where you found it. This is obviously important to every person who has a visual impairment, rather than placing things helter-skelter and having to search for them, wasting valuable time.

Of course, the woodshop teacher's lesson is true for all people, regardless of their vision status or station in life. But for the visually impaired it is imperative.

Typing class was an integral part of the curriculum at the blind school, beginning in the fifth grade, age 11. Typing gave me the means to complete homework and communicate with teachers in the public school system who were not trained to work with the visually impaired and people who used braille. It allowed me to transfer from the blind school to public school and become the first blind child to enroll in the Zanesville public school system. And it turned out to be especially useful once computer technology became so dominant, with so many advantages for blind people. More on that later.

Still, in all my years at the blind school, I never stopped dreaming of attending public school in Zanesville and returning full time to my home and family there.

Chapter 3: Back in Zanesville and Public School

And at the end of the seventh grade, my dream came true, and I transferred from the blind school to the public school system in Zanesville! This became possible mainly due to the efforts of my mother, bless her heart, and another rather remarkable person, an osteopath practicing in Zanesville, a blind man also, who happened to be on the school board and lobbied for my return.

Now I was able to forget the travel, the being away from home. And most importantly, I was able to establish myself as the first blind person to attend public school in Zanesville, giving me full-time contact with the sighted world as an eighth-grader at Roosevelt Junior High.

I was ready for public school, but public school wasn't really ready for me.

When I entered Roosevelt, there was no way for me to obtain a braille English book, for example. Braille's expense wasn't in the school board's budget. Only one or two places in America made braille textbooks, most of them by a company in Louisville. But they would only create braille books that large numbers of people would use; they wouldn't "braille" a book for a single student.

So that was a problem: I couldn't get any of the textbooks in braille.

Luckily, I had several dedicated student volunteers who were willing to read assigned lessons and class activities to me. All those volunteers were friends and good students, and their goodness rubbed off on me. God bless them.

Today, blind schools have special classes in public school systems and make talking computer technology and other resources available to blind students. That makes learning a lot easier than it was in my day, in the fifties.

We had no adaptation except utilizing the typewriter, and one was made available to me. Even tape recorders at that time, the big old bulky reel-to-reel types, were in their infancy.

So school was tough, but life in the neighborhood with my friends was a blast. I had a lot of fun and adventures in junior high and high school in Zanesville. One day I remember, not long after returning home for good, we went to a movie that featured a race car jumping up and ramp and through a ring of fire, ending in a crash landing.

Of course, when we got home, someone had the bright idea that we should build a ramp and try to recreate the stunt, fire and all, on our bicycles. Our ramp was pretty ramshackle, and we lit the fire, and several kids went flying over the flames successfully. I, of course, decided that I should try to do this, too, and to the hoots and "Go for it!" calls of my small crowd of playmates, I took my bike back several yards from the ramp and prepared to go. I approached where I thought the ramp was, pedaling my ass off, but nothing happened—I wasn't catapulted into the air. I'd missed the whole damn thing.

This was hilarious not only to me but was doubly so to my onlooking pals. They celebrated my mishap with hoots of derision and calls of "Attaboy, Jim!" Needless to say, I demanded another attempt and did, that time, hit the ramp, fly over the fire, and land on my wheels, thus becoming the only flying blind kid in the neighborhood.

I remember attending a picnic at a local lake, celebrating the end of ninth grade and our impending entry into high school. We had the whole day to swim, sunbathe, and enjoy the lake and park grounds. Someone had decided the night before that the picnic would taste better with a little beer and had stashed some in the cool waters of the lake the night before.

Long story short, seven or eight of us were enjoying our picnic lunch and our beer by ourselves, away from the bulk of the student body, when a park employee, seeing us where we shouldn't have been, stopped his truck to see what we were doing. We said we were eating lunch when I proceeded to knock over a beer, which ran all over the picnic table. Beer, as we all know, does not resemble soda.

At our return to the school, we were herded into the principal's office, where the irate principal and teachers confronted us. Threats were made to demote us or not pass us through to the tenth grade. Other admonishments were piled upon us, and our parents were called. After the furor died down, we were told how worthless we were and that we were probably on our way to reform school. Nothing ever came of it, and most of us involved turned into fine, upstanding citizens.

As I said earlier, one of my strong suits was music. The music department at Zanesville High during my years there was staffed by very talented musician-teachers. The drama club and the music department would get together every spring to produce and perform well-known musicals such as *Oklahoma* and *South Pacific*, to mention a couple.

For *Oklahoma* and *South Pacific*, I played in the orchestra and memorized the scores so that I wouldn't make the music sound too modern through improvisation. My senior year the production was the hit musical *Plain and Fancy*. I was chosen to be a role player in that production, playing Papa Yoder. As I said, the directing staff was highly skilled and passed that on to the student actors and actresses.

We earned great reviews, one of which came from the drama department at Ohio State. During the same year we did *Oklahoma* at Zanesville High, so did the university in Columbus. Several of the actors and singers in the Ohio State production of *Oklahoma* attended our performance in Zanesville and apparently told our production people that our show was even better than theirs! That came as high praise, and of course I was pleased to be a part of it, playing clarinet in the orchestra.

There is such a thing as braille music sheets. The problem is, obviously, that it is impossible to read braille music and play your instrument at the same time. You can learn the piece from braille, but it still requires memorization. When I was a member of the band at the blind school, each chair in the band memorized his part in the score. The director would find time to teach each part to the respective group of musicians. Then we'd put it together in practice.

When I was playing in Zanesville High's orchestra, I'd memorize my piece—and others' parts—by listening. Sometimes, I'm sure, my rendition gave the music a more modern flavor than the score indicated, but for the most part I was able to stick to the music as written and didn't modernize too much.

Other students in the formal bands I played in accepted me as I presented myself and would help me if I asked them. But they usually left me on my own to work it out.

My senior year in high school, I was chosen to be part of the All-Ohio Youth Choir, which met and performed with other vocal students from different parts of the state. We met at Wilmington College and spent weekends rehearsing. That activity culminated in a concert accompanied by an orchestra of all-star college students. We presented our show at the college gymnasium. Of course, I was the only blind person involved, and most of the students didn't even realize I couldn't see. There again my ability to acclimate to new physical surroundings served me well.

That was a lot of fun for me. And it proved to me that I was making an excellent adjustment of my disability to the public school world and Zanesville itself.

I seem to have a rather wild side of my personality, and it came out strongly during my public school years. I was willing to do things that bordered on delinquent behavior, I think to some degree to be accepted by my peer groups, who were mainly athletes and wild-eyed teenagers. But it was often a thrill and the adrenaline high seemed worth the risk.

I had an arrangement with several of my friends—Steve McGlade, for one. When it became necessary to run after doing something mischievous or illegal, I would place my hand on the back of their belt and take off with them. That allowed me to join my friends in fleeing the 'po (police) or just plain angry citizens.

This little trick came to be especially helpful when enraged drivers stopped their cars and chased after us. Why? Because we'd been throwing water balloons or snowballs—depending on the season—at them.

This manner of escape—my hand on a buddy's belt—made for very effective getaways.

One trick I'll never forget involved placing a lawn chair in the middle of the street. After borrowing a chair from a neighbor's front porch, we proceeded to tie one end of a long rope to the chair and toss the other end over the power line. Then we took that loose line and ran up onto a nearby hillside to see things develop.

When a driver approached, he'd stop and get out of the car to move the chair out of the way. Then we'd all pull on the other end of the rope, out of sight, and lift the chair, leaving it suspended over the head of the bewildered driver, and causing all of us on the hillside to break into a round of hoarse laughs.

I'd hear the car stop, the door open, the man's steps on the street, occasionally a "What the hell?" or "You assholes" once they saw the chair pulled up above the car. That was funny. It didn't hurt anyone.

One time a driver got so annoyed that he began to chase us. Everyone took off, me with my hand on Steve's belt. We ran between two houses when we were suddenly pitched forward into the air after tripping over and falling across a knee-high fence that Steve didn't see. Him first and me right after him since, of course, I was unaware of it!

Luckily the driver had stopped chasing us before this happened, or we probably would have been caught and punished.

Another time, something that became folklore for our group as we aged, we "borrowed" potato chips from the truck that supplied area stores with snacks. At night the truck was parked in the neighborhood in front of the driver's home. One night, coming home from a high school game, we "borrowed" some chips from the truck and enjoyed them for several weeks, having stashed them in an old, abandoned barn nearby that we used as a hideout.

We also used to steal beer from unsuspecting neighbors who used to store it on their back porches to keep cold. One friend, Chick, was a paper carrier in the area, and he knew which homes kept beer on their porches. He'd tell us where the beer was, and we'd visit them at night to "borrow" the beer and stash it—along with the chips—in our hideout. Beer and chips made a great combination for teenaged troublemakers.

One night we were tipped off that a neighbor who owned a nearby bar had a case of whisky in his garage. We borrowed the case of whisky and stashed it under some brush near Zanesville High. We probably ultimately would have ended up in real trouble over that situation, but one of our group blabbed to an older student, who, in turn, borrowed the whisky from us and sold it in the neighborhood as moonshine. We probably didn't need to drink the whisky—or sell it, either, which may have ended us in real trouble with the 'po—so theft upon theft at that time probably worked out well for us.

We were pretty harmless, all in all. We didn't steal money, didn't do vandalism. Beer and potato chips was about as far as we would go.

My hearing came in handy to my fellow miscreants. I've always had great hearing, and I'm sure, I use it differently from a sighted person. When a sighted person hears a noise, he can look to see where the noise came from. I can't do that, so I need to be able to locate the source of the sounds without being able to see it.

A lifetime of necessity has worked my hearing into a highly reliable sense, and as I do use it differently, I can hear certain sounds which, to a sighted person, are unnoticeable.

For instance, when I was a kid and my hearing was better than it is now, I could tell whether the radio or TV was on because the TVs at those times had a very high-pitched squeal that the radio didn't.

I don't hear it now, and I don't know whether that's because my hearing is worse or that TVs are designed better, but that's one of the first things that I remember hearing that others couldn't.

The way I use my hearing, when I hear a noise, I usually know what it is and where it is without being able to look. That just comes from practice and memory and being able to remember what the sound I hear is.

Because of hearing skills, I became the lookout—or better, the "hear-out"—for some of our nefarious activities.

I'd hear things they wouldn't, maybe because they were concentrating visually in whatever they were doing: doors opening, latches opening or closing. I was so acutely able to do that, that they'd trust me to warn them if anyone was approaching.

Here again, I got involved with a lot of that stuff just to show people that I could be...normal. I didn't do it because I had larceny in my heart; I wasn't a born John Dillinger or anything like that. You know, a lot of peer pressure. I started smoking because of peer pressure—as a Boy Scout! Kept that bad habit for twelve years.

Some of my friends liked to look in on teenage girls at night when they were getting ready for bed and neglected to close their blinds. They were never challenged, so I can't say that it was due to my acute hearing or just dumb luck.

Willits was one of my more adventurous buddies. One day he was bent on borrowing a car in the neighborhood. He knew that the car owner always left his car unlocked, parked in the garage. Many cars back in the early fifties still had an on/off switch for the motor, so you didn't need a key if the door was left unlocked. Buick was still making cars with the on/off switch.

When Willits and I were thirteen or so, he borrowed a car in the early morning hours and drove it over to my house. We had a big old garage, built around 1925, with a slate roof, off the back alley, away from the house. On the side of the garage hung a big wooden ladder. Willits took the ladder down and positioned it beneath my second-story bedroom window.

I climbed down, and off we went on a joy ride through town. After a while Willits drove me back home, where I climbed back up to my bedroom. Willits returned the ladder to its place on the side of the garage and returned the car to its owner, no one in either house any the wiser.

Other times I went with him on foot and stood nearby as hearout as he boosted a car for a joy ride.

We didn't get caught, thank God, with car theft being a serious infraction, of course. In fact, later on Willits grabbed a car on his own, wrecked it, and then stole another one to get home. He was lucky to not get caught or hurt. I decided then that car theft was out of my league and never attempted it again in the future.

Luckily my parents didn't find out about my hoodlum ways, and I'm certainly glad for that. My mother would have killed me, being, as she was, a very honorable and churchgoing lady.

My only scrape with the law occurred not in Zanesville but in Coshocton, a town about thirty miles to the north. Coshocton High came to Zanesville one Friday night when I was a junior to play our football team and after the game groups of partisans from both sides exchanged rude words, each side threatening to kick the other's ass and such.

Coshocton was big rival of Zanesville's in the midfifties, part of a strong Central Ohio League that also included high school teams from Cambridge, Newark, Lancaster, Chillicothe, Dover, and New Philadelphia.

Anyway, we thought it would be a good idea to meet these guys back in Coshocton and show them who's boss. So about fifteen of us piled into six cars and drove up there, about thirty miles north of Zanesville, where it turns out the police were waiting for our arrival. They intercepted our cars, then invited us down to the station to talk, they said. At that point, they decided to confiscate our beer and herd us into a big holding cell.

As we sat there stewing, I remember leading the boys in a song:

> If I had the wings of an angel
> Over these prison walls we would fly

At some point, I really needed to use the can, which was outside the holding cell, so I pounded on the door and told the officer through the peephole that I needed to go, no kidding. I told him I was blind and that he needed to take me over there in a hurry, one of those situations.

I think he saw that he would have his hands full with a blind kid he'd have to take to the bathroom every few minutes, so about fifteen minutes later, they cut us loose. We were probably in there a couple of hours. They didn't arrest us, didn't take our names, didn't call our parents, just let us go. We left Coshocton immediately.

I was always strong for my age and size as a kid and as a teenager. Starting in my sophomore year in high school, I began to participate in weight lifting and other activities to build my strength. I began doing push-ups on a daily basis. At first, I did fifteen push-ups three times a day, ultimately building that up to one hundred push-ups three times a day. I got pretty strong, I have to say.

There again, I think I did this to show that even though I was blind, I could stand out in physical activity. With this reputation as a strong guy, I was never picked on by bullies too much as a high schooler and later in life.

I did wrestle for a short time at the Zanesville Y and had some limited success. I was never pinned, but I had other fish to fry and didn't stick with it, so my career as a wrestler was brief. I think I would have been very good since I was strong and quick on my feet.

Later in life, some friends gave me the nickname Big Cat since I had great balance. I was usually able to maintain, or regain, my balance in certain precarious situations while walking. For example, if I unexpectedly stepped off a street curb, I was always able to regain my balance before my face hit the pavement.

I had a fairly good social life with the opposite sex during junior high and high school and later in college. I must have been okay looking since many very nice young ladies consented to be my date.

I lost my virginity when I was a junior in high school due to the promiscuity of one of the young ladies in our class, not that I was extremely handsome and charming. But I was glad to get that out of the way and at least be equal to many of my classmates and friends who had beat me to the punch, so to speak, with the ladies.

My years in high school actually flew by. Three years seemed to come and go in an instant, especially in retrospect. I'll never forget walking across the stage at graduation and shaking hands with the dignitaries in attendance—the principal of the high school, the dean of boys, the area superintendent, and most importantly, the blind osteopath who helped make it possible for me to attend Zanesville High and experience that final success. I'll never forget my reaction when everyone shook my hand, and he, the doctor, told me how proud he was of my school performance.

While many of my classmates were rejoicing—smiling, laughing, and joking—I was in tears, knowing that this important part of my life was finally over. I had overcome many challenges with the help and support of my family and friends and was ready to move onto the next chapter in my life.

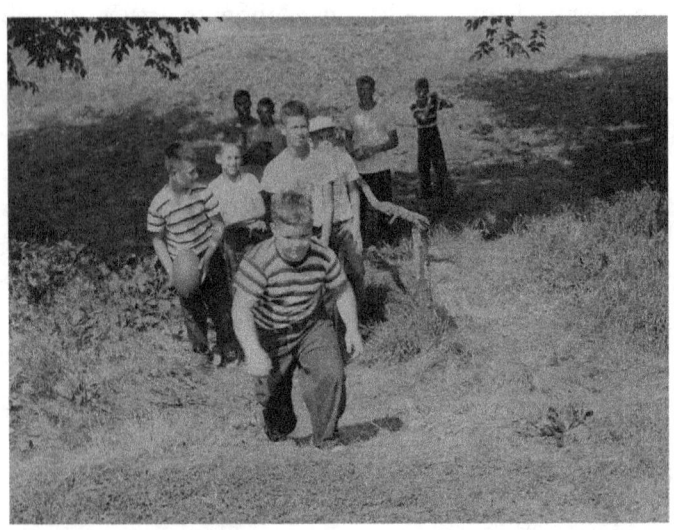

Jim leading a group of fellow campers up a hill at Camp Moores.

But what the hell was that chapter? This was a new situation. I didn't know which way to go. I had completed the structured life of American secondary education, and now what? What's available for a blind man in terms of supporting himself and, if he's lucky, a family in later life? This was back in the day when blind people still sat on corners looking blind and selling pencils and newspapers.

Most of my good friends we planning on going onto the next step—college! I hadn't thought about that. Wow! Talk about fucking panic! I started drinking a little bit more than usual. I didn't know exactly what to do with my time. One of my friends—Jack, for whom I would later be best man at his wedding and a friend until his death—told me about YMCA Camp Moores on the banks of the Muskingum just north of town. I had attended camp when I was a kid as a camper, but not as a staff member. I didn't think of that, but the more we talked about it, I decided that working at the camp would be fun and a maybe a good way to open new roads for me.

I went and talked to Howard Miller, the boys' secretary of the YMCA in Zanesville, and persuaded him into hiring me for a small job at the camp that summer. I was to be the music director. I would lead singing and songs after meals, at campfires, and during evening activities. I got room and board and $15 a week. I decided to do that and opened a new relationship with an old friend—Camp Moores, where I had spent three summers as a camper, a total of twelve weeks, back in the late forties and early fifties.

My new job turned out to be a great experience. I had good relationships with the other staff and with the kids. They accepted me and my disability, and most of them, I'm sure, after a while didn't even think of me as being disabled. I would pitch softball to them, lead songs, of course, and other activities during evening campfires and meetings. I swam with them, canoed with them, and even, after learning the rules myself, helped demonstrate canoe safety. I was a staff member on many canoe trips on the Muskingum and surrounding rivers, including the Walhonding and the Tuscarawas.

Later I would canoe on other rivers in other states with groups of men, and this certainly laid a good foundation and gave me a workable knowledge of canoe skills and safety requirements.

My friend Jack and I talked at length about paddling a canoe from Zanesville on the Muskingum, to the Ohio River and then south on the Mississippi to New Orleans. We set up a timetable, even including some short stops in bars we'd see along the way, since we both liked to drink some. Unfortunately, time never allowed us to do that, and now, of course, I'm too old to think about it. Maybe that will be on my bucket list for the next life, ha ha!

Joe, one of my closest friends, talked to me a lot after high school about going on to college. Joe was not only a great friend, but he actually worried about me as a person and what was going to happen to me in the long run. He kept saying, "Come on, go to college with us!" He and another classmate, Andy, who at an earlier age had loaned me his bicycle to learn how to ride, decided that they would attend Ohio State in Columbus. And they thought I should go with them. But I didn't, at least not right away.

They enrolled in September of 1958. That left me alone in Zanesville, knocking around on my own, once in a while spending time with Jack and Scott, another good friend, drinking a lot of suds and once in a while getting involved with a bar girl or two.

That first summer after graduating from high school, I wrote my first song while working at camp. I composed another song or two, just because I had more time to devote to it. Anyway, summer became fall and fall became winter, as it always does, and Joe and Andy both worked on me during trips home. Finally, I decided to consider college.

I contacted the Rehabilitation Service Commission in the Ohio Bureau of Service to the Blind for help in paying college fees. BSB had helped me during junior high and especially high school in the form of money to pay readers thirty-five cents an hour to read lessons and assignments to me.

Chapter 4: Ohio State

With Joe's help, I applied to Ohio State and was accepted to enroll in winter quarter, January of 1959. Oh shit, another break from home. Another situation in which I'd have to leave home and live on my own again.

It wasn't a hell of a lot easier to me at this time, even though I was eleven years older than when I first entered the blind school. It was still difficult.

I remember my mother and brother Ken dropping me off at Stradley Hall, a brand-new dormitory at that time, on Eleventh Avenue in OSU's south campus. I shed a few tears, it's true, even though I was kind of embarrassed about it. It was scary, it was. I knew I was good, I knew I could take care of myself, but here I was learning a new geographic situation.

To make matters worse, about a month before leaving for Ohio State, I broke a bone in my foot playing football. The ball of my foot was split in half, and the doctors couldn't do anything to set the bone. I just had to walk on the foot carefully until it healed. And that's how I entered college, limping to class.

Joe, now deceased, and other friends spent time helping me learn the enormous campus. When I got my class schedule just before the start of each quarter, they would take me around campus to the different buildings where my classes were. After one or two circuits of the new route, I could get to class and home again independently, usually without any help.

I carry a white cane now, but I didn't use one at Ohio State. I walked through the OSU campus—one of the nation's largest—relying solely on echolocation, memory, and landmarks.

Getting Around: Echolocation, Memory, Landmarks

Blind people use different abilities to help us travel about on our own. It's kind of hard to explain because it's first nature to us. It's what we do. I relied most heavily on my echolocation skills and my memory, and I also kept track of the placement of permanent landmarks, for lack of a better term.

For instance, in walking down a sidewalk, I may come upon a large object that I pick up using echolocation—a tree, a lamppost, a retaining wall. I make a mental note of that for the next trip to the same destination.

When I was living that first quarter in Stradley Hall, I'd leave the dorm for my first class—in University Hall just north of the Oval—and immediately turn right onto a big cement sidewalk, a walkway that I took over to Twelfth Avenue, along Baker Hall. At Twelfth Avenue, there was a crosswalk. I knew then that I was at Twelfth when I heard the traffic. So I'm picking up cues, mainly the flow of traffic, the voices of other people alongside me talking, or the sounds of their shoes slowing or stopping, as we all converged on the crosswalk.

I remember there was a slight slope in the sidewalk as it met the curb. You learn to remember to be aware of all these things. Memory, of course, is key in all this. So when I began to cross Twelfth Avenue, as soon as I stepped down, I heard the echo of the curb I just stepped over. Ironically, hearing a curb using echolocation is harder now than it was in my day because of the curb cuts to help wheelchair users, which came about as a result of the 1991 Americans with Disabilities Act.

Later, when I was working in Wisconsin, I was a member of the Governor's Committee on Disabilities. One of the things we worked on, and I think the ADA writers may have used it as a model in crafting their legislation, was the importance of using difference surfaces in the curb cuts. You notice that when you get to a curb cut the surface may be a bit rougher—like corduroy or like gravel in concrete—to warn blind people that they're approaching a corner and they should stop and assess the situation and not walk right out into the street.

Unfortunately, many curb cuts still today have no surface changes to alert blind people that they're at the corner, so we have to take note of the sudden slope from sidewalk to street level, another thing to remember.

We didn't have curb cuts at Ohio State at the time, of course, so I had to detect the curb, up or down with echolocation. I learned all this by traveling the campus, first with Joe, then on my own. So as I went through south campus to the Oval, one way to go took me through an area called the hollow, near Mirror Lake. It had paths like a wheel with spokes going out. I'd come to an intersection, and the spokes would go out in different directions. So I had to learn, and remember, which spoke went to which location.

That's true in the Oval too. (*The OSU Oval is a huge green space, crossed with many paths in all directions, that runs from the main library on Neil Avenue east almost to High Street, the university's eastern limit.*) I learned from friends and from experience that the walkways crossing the Oval also went in every direction, again, kind of like spokes on a wheel but a bit more complicated. In the middle of the Oval sat a large wooden information booth. That was another landmark I relied on, using echolocation from the hard heels on my shoes. The sound bouncing off the booth helped orient me to the direction and sidewalk I needed to be on to get to my class.

I figured out how to navigate it just from memory and sense of direction that I was blessed with. And OSU wasn't as big then as it is now. Classes were mostly around the Oval and Neil Avenue, and some buildings north of the Oval.

At one point on the route I often took, there was a telephone pole right before I got to the curb. I know it was there because I heard its echo. So then I knew I was almost at the curb. Landmarks can be many different things, a brick walkway for example. There was a brick walkway in front of the administration building, which was between Derby Hall and University Hall. If I came across the North Oval in front of Derby Hall, I'd know to turn left and then cross the street, and the next block would be the administration building with the brick sidewalk.

Of course, if there was snow on the ground, it would muffle the distinctive sound of feet on brick or cement, and I'd have to rely to an even greater degree on my echolocation.

After the next crosswalk, about half a block farther, I'd come to University Hall with cement steps and large buttresses on either side. The buttresses offered good cues for my echolocation, and then I'd know that I was nearing the steps to enter the building.

Once inside University Hall, I remembered that there were twenty-three steps from the first floor to the second floor. A lot of people think I counted steps to get around in general, but I never did that on flat ground. I will, however, count steps going up or down a flight of stairs. For example, I know that I have fifteen steps to go from the main floor in my house up to the second-floor bedrooms. Counting stair steps helps avoid jerking the hell out of my leg if I miscalculate, something that sighted people tell me happens to them, too, in the dark or if they're not paying attention. It's not foolproof; once in a while I'd forget and maybe miss a step. But here again is where good sense of balance comes in, so I never fell or anything.

Once up to the right floor in University Hall, I had to know which way to turn to get to my classroom. Then I'd find the door using echolocation, go inside, and then find an empty chair to sit in. Of course, as I said earlier, my friends helped me find the best routes—outside and inside—before classes began to help orient me around campus. It sounds difficult and complicated, but with the skills I had developed over the years and with my friends' initial assistance, it wasn't that hard, and I was able to travel independently around campus.

So in terms of getting around, it's memory, it's use of echolocation, it's use of landmarks, surfaces—they all come into play. Building memory skills is essential for blind people. I think that most visually impaired people I have known have developed their memories to a far greater degree than sighted people, as long as they didn't have other developmental disabilities.

It's easily explained: we can't readily take notes, write things down, use visual cues. We have to remember addresses, phone numbers, credit card numbers—the list goes on. Those of us blind people with higher than average intelligence can remember more because we've trained ourselves—on a daily basis over the span of our lifetimes—to do so. And our memories may include unusual things. I can remember how to get from one place to another, regardless of what state we're in, as long as I've been there before and was made familiar with the route the first time. It's actually no more glamorous than that.

It's just based on the fact that we must, so we do. For some reason, I'm just better at it than the average bear.

I was reluctant to use a white cane during my years at Ohio State because I didn't want to be considered different, I wanted to be able to do it all by myself, to show people that I wasn't much different from them.

The white cane, a long white stick with a red tip, familiar to most of the public, is a very important travel aid to the blind and visually impaired and is recognized internationally as such. It is a visual communication to anyone who sees it that the user is blind, but it can be used to produce tapping noises useful to those of us using echolocation. It also can be used as a "feeler" to find curbs and other landmarks if hearing is clouded by noise or other distractions.

Some blind people use guide dogs, also well-known to the public. These dogs are trained by experts to lead a blind person, who gives the dog verbal directions to follow. In this way, the dog becomes the eyes for the blind owner. But the dog is not a user's mind, so a blind person with a dog must already be a fairly independent traveler to give a guide dog the proper commands to reach one's destination. In other words, you can't just tell the dog, "I want to go to the barbershop." You have to know where the barbershop is before getting underway. Say the shop is the fourth door on the left from the corner of First and Main. Once at the corner, you'd give the dog the command, "In," which tells him that you want to find the first door. But you need the fourth door, so you'd give him the command four times in succession—once for each door the dog stops in front of—until you reach the barbershop. As in the case of the white cane, the sight of a dog in harness tells the sighted public that the person holding the dog's handle is visually impaired.

If I did get confused traveling around campus—which didn't happen often, thank God—all I had to do was ask, and most people were friendly enough to realize that I didn't have good vision. Many of them thought I had partial vision the way I was getting around. And they were glad to help.

People were amazed at my skills. I was never amazed because to me it came naturally. I accepted it as part of my life as a blind person, not knowing at the time that I was doing things that perhaps other blind people didn't normally do.

Now there were a few times where I got confused and no one was around. Believe it or not, I got myself back on track by listening for the bells ringing from Orton Hall on the south side of the Oval. I wonder if they still ring those bells? Those bells became a travel cue for me, especially in my initial orientation on campus. The bells rang every fifteen minutes, so if I really got off track, I'd wait to hear the damn bell to tell me where I was, to give me an idea. I'd hear it, figure out which direction I appeared to be from it, and then I'd go on my way.

In this way, I traveled to and from my dorm room on South Campus and, later, from the fraternity house off-campus a mile or more each way to get to classes. From the frat, I had to negotiate even busier street crossings—including Indianola Avenue and High Street, Columbus's main north-south thoroughfare—of course, at traffic lights wherever available.

Back to the classroom. Unfortunately, college in the late fifties and early sixties was no more oriented for blind people than high school was.

To remember lectures, I bought what was euphemistically called a "portable" tape recorder. The idea was to take it to class to record lectures. That idea didn't last long at all. The damn thing was supposed to be portable, but it must have weighed twenty pounds. Then I had to find a place to plug it in, no batteries involved, in the classrooms. That was a pain. Then upon lugging the thing back to my room, I had to listen again to the professor's lecture. That ended up taking up more time than I had available. I'd go to class, record the class, then listen to the lecture again later on tape.

It didn't work for me, so I fell back again on using personal readers. I'd have the instructor ask anyone in the class if they'd be interested in helping me by reading textbooks and sharing their notes with me. Bless their hearts, I was always able to find skilled, smart people to help.

That obviously helped me, and it helped them review the material too—killed two birds with one stone. It was mostly girls in the education classes I took. And they were glad to do it. Women were more apt to help, and I made some good friends that way, too. Some girlfriends, but mostly just platonic scholars trying to do our best. Get your work done and go home.

I was fortunate, too, that my brother Bob and his family had just returned to Ohio from Massachusetts about the same time I entered OSU, settling in Columbus to work for Nationwide Insurance. He read textbooks to me a lot, and I taped our sessions in his house over by Riverside Hospital, about three miles from OSU, so that I could go over it again later if I wanted to.

It was really cool, and he'd read everything like a radio announcer, like he was back working on air as a journalist. I remember I researched a paper on economic geography that focused on the economics of the Muskingum Valley, relying mostly on material written by a guy I had at Zanesville High as an English teacher. He was also an area historian, and I used a lot of his books as reference material. I recorded it, and Bob typed it up—hell, it was the only A+ I ever got in my life!

There were organizations available in the country at the time, one specifically called Recording for the Blind, which was dedicated to recording textbooks on tape, later on floppy disks, so that blind students could at least listen to the assigned books.

However, Recording for the Blind was set up to provide services to college students on a semester basis. But Ohio State at that time was on a quarter system. Three quarters equaled two semesters during the September to June school year, so the quarters were shorter. Because of that, I was usually behind since the books were recorded in installments fit for semesters. I used the recorded material when available, but I was usually behind in my reading since the installments often arrived later than when I needed them. It caused me a hell of a lot of stress as a student. I was always behind.

Somehow, I got through by listening in class and using the student readers when possible.

My main way of preparing for approaching tests, in high school and early in college, was to just sit myself down and go over everything in my head.

Once I declared as an education major, a lot of us in the same classes would organize study groups and discuss what we thought would be on the tests. That was another way I got through.

I had to listen in class the whole time—that's how I'd absorb the material—and I'd fall asleep a lot. I got accused several times when I wasn't sleeping because I didn't wear glasses. I'd sit there with my eyes closed, but I'd be awake. I got accused two or three times from pissed-off profs. I'd get indignant too—damn it, I wasn't asleep! So I listened in class, had people read to me, and went over other students' notes with them. I'm surprised I made it through, truthfully.

Instead of written tests, I'd take oral exams, usually administered by the professor. It's hard to bullshit through an oral exam, and I was lucky to make it through. It was arduous and precarious at best.

Talk about butterflies and sleepless nights! I still have what I call "stress dreams," based on my days at Ohio State and the feeling I had of always feeling behind and ill-prepared.

During my second quarter at OSU, I made contact with some blind guys I had attended the Blind School with many moons before. They were all living together in Columbus near the campus, and I reestablished friendships with them. Also living in the area was Joy, a girl who had also been in my class at the blind school. She was now a buxom nineteen-year-old and looked pretty good. I began a relationship with her and damn near flunked out that quarter because I was paying more attention to her and her willing body than I did to my schoolwork.

At some point, Joe sat me down and talked turkey to me, as a best friend will. I maintained the relationship with Joy but put it in better perspective and set some priorities. That affair lasted for several quarters, but ended when I decided that our relationship was getting too serious. I didn't need a love commitment at that point in my life.

Later at OSU, while walking home from class, I ran into a girl from Zanesville who I had been in social dancing classes with back in the eighth and ninth grades. She attended the Catholic high school in Zanesville, but after asking her out for coffee, and later that week on a drinking date, we established a relationship which lasted until she graduated later that year.

You may wonder: what makes women sexy to a blind man? The most prevalent feature, as you might imagine, is her voice. That is equivalent to what sighted men experience in their first vision of a woman. If a lady has a pleasant attractive voice, it goes a long way in forming your initial impression.

However, that is not always accurate. In fact, gauging a woman's attractiveness solely on her voice can be highly inaccurate. It has happened to me—and to other blind male friends I've talked to—that, after hearing a woman's voice, I would think, "Well, that's an attractive gal," and later find out that the voice in question actually belonged to a man!

Other times, a pleasant, sexy voice can be attached to people who are physically unattractive to those with vision. But the voice is the first dominant impression.

Of course, what women say, how they say it, their manner overall, is important in forming impressions beyond the music of their voices alone. Their manner may be coquettish or completely unemotional or a dozen other things. All of them factor in to give you a fuller idea of the person.

Looking back on my scholastic career on campus, it seems that I was fortunate to have what I see now as understanding instructors. I think they realized that I was trying my ass off. Oftentimes they'd give me that benefit of the doubt when it came to a sketchy answer or a stumbling recital. I don't know how I ever got through freshman

English. I suspect that the themes that we were assigned every week or so went unread by the instructor.

I can only think this because at that time I had a hard time spelling *cat*, since most of my life material was read to me rather than reading it myself. Most sighted people learn to spell by reading words in print, and I didn't have that advantage. Anyway, I got through freshman English by the skin of my butt, and other English courses I took during my college career didn't require theme writing.

Every quarter at Ohio State meant learning new buildings, new classrooms, parts of the huge campus that were strange to me. But with Joe's help, mainly, in acclimating me to my new surroundings and paths needed to get there, I managed. Joe was my roommate then; later we would be fraternity brothers.

I lucked out several times, especially in terms of required courses. Freshman math was mandatory at that time, but I talked with the head of the math department, and he determined that my major didn't really require math. So he excused me from that. Later I changed majors to escape the requirement of taking a foreign language, also a scary, almost impossible, subject—to me anyway.

Phi Gamma Delta

My brother Ken also attended Ohio State and graduated the quarter before I began. He had me as a guest to his Phi Gamma Delta fraternity house for a few days in fall quarter before I enrolled, and I met a lot of the guys there. They saw me operate as a disabled person, saw my skills in travel and in acclimating to new places. That experience, I'm sure, paved the way for me to be invited to pledge the fraternity during my first quarter.

Joe and I were roommates in the dorm, and we all pledged Phi Gamma Delta, which was one of the better-known fraternities on campus. For me, a fraternity was an island in the sea of forty thousand or so students at Ohio State. It gave me instant access to friendships, social functions, and a feeling of belonging—an important social requirement for a disabled person.

A lot of disabled people become isolated simply because it's hard to initiate relationships. Think about it. What's the first thing most people do when they meet someone: you look at their eyes, their faces, to gauge reactions to you and record initial feelings. Blind people do not have that advantage. We have to operate on what we hear, the way we are talked to and gut feelings. At least, that's how I have operated, and it's worked for me through my life.

Phi Gamma Delta not only functioned as a fraternity, with parties, social happenings, but we also were active in community projects. We helped raise funds for deserving enterprises, and we volunteered at community centers and soup kitchens and attempted to be good citizens—within reason.

We were known as a social fraternity, with the emphasis on *social*. There was a party every week, whether you wanted to attend it or not. They usually included live music, dancing, and, of course, beer—or what they used to call "barley pop" in Wisconsin. I had an enormous appetite for barley pop and soon developed a reputation for being able to hold my beer. With Friday being the last day of the class week for most of us, it meant a little bit of barley pop after class or after initiating the "TGIF-ing," which meant going drinking on Friday afternoon instead of going to class.

Friday night dinners at the fraternity were informal, rather than coat and tie, which was the rule Monday through Thursday. One Friday we gathered for dinner with spaghetti and meatballs, garlic bread, the whole nine yards. On that night, following rounds of afternoon drinking by many of us, the dining hall exploded into an impromptu food fight. It developed into a real melee and quickly spread from the dining room into the lounge upstairs and beyond.

It was a real mess, and it pissed me off, too, since I was hungry and the spaghetti and meatballs our cook prepared was excellent. I grabbed my plate and retired to the underside of one of the tables, where I quickly swallowed my dinner without too much interference from the battlers. But what a mess! It took professional cleaners to come in and finally put the house back in order. I think we only did that once.

One custom in the fraternity was to give a brother a fully clothed shower if he became "pinned" to his lady, meaning engaged to be engaged. The notion was that she would consent to be your girl throughout college and then maybe your wife thereafter.

Earlier the custom had been to pitch a brother into Mirror Lake, an overgrown puddle at the south edge of campus. But since the lake stank of sulfur at the time, this practice was soon outlawed by the university.

The active pinner was expected to resist getting thrown in the shower. One day it was my turn for the shower after being pinned to a gal. I was pretty husky at that time, and strong to boot, having worked out for years with weights and doing push-ups, so when the pledge class attacked me, I resisted mightily. The mass of us swarmed throughout the dining room, overturning tables and chairs.

Every time someone laid his hands on me, I'd throw two or three of them together, yelling "Gotcha!" The house mother who witnessed the brawl told me later that it was the first time in her memory that any newly pinned member successfully resisted getting thrown in the shower. I never got wet that night, and my reputation as a scrapper spread.

When I was a sophomore, several of my fraternity brothers convinced me that I could make a successful skydive. They had already lined up a trial jump at a local airport near Columbus. I figured that since I had good balance, had wrestled and knew how to fall, that I should try it. Well, I was never so scared in my life. Looking back, I would probably never do it again.

Today, blind people skydive either by being talked down by walkie-talkies or by jumping in tandem with an instructor. Frankly, I'm still surprised that I was even allowed to participate by the skydiving facility. Probably today a blind skydiver jumping alone for the first time wouldn't be allowed. But I lucked out and came through with no injuries and wasn't frightened to death. But if I were to go up again, the plane would have to be ready to crash before I'd jump out and pull the parachute!

Life in the frat was not always serious, obviously. Sleeping arrangements in the house were several. You could have your bed in a single or shared room or in a large unheated room called the dormitory. The dormitory was a large attic-type room with no heat, few windows, and a wooden floor.

Sometimes brothers who slept close to a window would wake up with snow on their blankets. Guys put more clothes on to go to bed than they wore during the daytime.

The buzzword in this story is *wooden floor*, which was not only cold to bare feet but very receptive to vibrations. If one were to place a household appliance like, say, a large Hoover vacuum cleaner on it, the floor would vibrate like hell.

Of course, most of the brothers wouldn't have thought up such a stunt. They would have needed light from the hallway to see what they were doing. However, that light would have woken up brothers trying to sleep and killed the whole deal.

I, however, required no light to quietly place the offending vacuum cleaner in an appropriately noisy spot. And I figured out that if I turned the switch to On before setting the cleaner down, I could be out of the area by the time I plugged it in some twenty feet away.

I would sneak the vacuum cleaner into the dorm, set it down just right, exit the room, plug in the machine, and then wait for the chaos to begin. The machine would bolt on, shaking the whole room awake to curses while I laughed out of hearing range.

One brother got so angry one night that he grabbed the vibrating cleaner, opened one of the few windows, and tossed it out to a loud crash on the street below.

But I went to the well once too often. One night, just as I placed the vacuum cleaner in a stealthy manner, everyone in the dorm greeted me. Caught red-handed! And red-faced. The laugh was on me, certainly, and laugh they did. It was funny enough for me to laugh too, especially when I learned that I wasn't going to be mauled by the brothers.

Since I was a good singer, I was involved in many of the musical activities of the fraternity, which were important in our social standing on campus. We would serenade sororities in the area and had several dinner parties for family members during the year. Those activities usually included some numbers from the fraternity glee club, of which I was a member.

Because of my singing talent and what I'm told were my good looks, I was chosen by my brothers to be the fraternity's candidate for "Golddigger King" of Greek Week in 1963. I competed with other so-called studs (which I never considered myself to be) from the other fraternities on campus. The top 10 candidates would travel around to the sororities on campus and ask for their votes. Unfortunately, I didn't make it to the top 10 cutoff, and for the first time in several years our fraternity was not represented in the voting.

In the following year's Greek Week talent show, I performed and took home second place. That got my name out as a talent, and I was invited to appear on a Columbus TV program called *The Jack Denton Show*. Soon after I began playing paying gigs around campus.

Another plus to being in the frat was that it provided me a steady supply of readers—pledges. Pledges had to do what you told them to, and reading to me was easy work for them, much better than cleaning toilets.

An even bigger thing the fraternity helped me with was passing tests. Through the years, brothers kept files of tests in several disciplines, with many of the tests being used quarter after quarter, year after year, for each new massive influx of freshmen and sophomores. These resources gave the user a pretty good chance of coming up with some of the test questions—and answers—prior to the test.

Since I was usually behind in my studies, due to the lack of available recorded books and other study aids for blind people at the time, I felt justified in taking advantage of any means available to improve my chances to get that all-important degree. Several of the test files I used to help me study were a great success—probably they were instrumental in getting me through.

One quarter, a fraternity brother in the same psychology class gave me the answers to a multiple choice test in advance. Because I took an oral test after written tests were administered to the sighted students, they had already taken the test and received the answers before I was called in for my oral exam. After my brother passed me the questions and answers, I then recorded the answers on braille cards that I concealed in my pocket. I passed the test easily, missing two questions on purpose to avoid drawing unwanted suspicion to my outstanding performance.

Another time, during a spring quarter, I avoided taking a final that I was unprepared for by telling the head of the department that I had the chance of a lifetime to work in a camp in northern Ontario, but that I had to report a week before the quarter was ending. He stated that since I had such a good mark in the class so far, he would give me the grade I had thus far, a B+ and give me permission to skip the final. Wow, saved my ass!

I'm not particularly proud of my unsavory conduct, but under the circumstances, I'd probably do it again to survive.

When I reached my final quarter at college, as an education major I was assigned to student-teach at Whetstone High in north Columbus, a few miles up the Olentangy River from OSU.

I had a great teacher-mentor at Whetstone. He was supportive and didn't seem to be doubtful at all of my ability to teach a senior class in Problems of Democracy. After he observed me for two or three periods, he left the classroom completely up to me and my own lesson plan.

I really had a great group of kids, too, which was apparent in many ways. As a student-teacher, I had a supervisor visit me in class at least once a week to monitor my performance and grade me.

The kids would always tip me off when the supervisor snuck into class. He usually didn't stay the full period, and when he left, of course, I could hear the door shut, but they would always let me know, "He's gone!" Then we would get back to the more informal, but effective, learning experience I had planned. I received a passing grade in student-teaching and earned my teaching license upon graduation.

One day during my last quarter at OSU, I was leaving for class after lunch at the fraternity, and some guys were playing basketball on our court in front of the house. I stopped for a second just to give them some grief, and one of them challenged me to take a shot. Mind you, I was behind a chest-high wall, some thirty feet from the basket. I said okay, they handed me the ball, and I took a jump shot from that distance. *Swish!* The ball never touched the rim! The guys damn near fainted, and so did I. I couldn't have done that again if I'd shot the ball all day. Talk about blind luck!

Anyway, I graduated from Ohio State in the spring of 1964. It was kind of an anticlimax. Many of my close friends in the frat house were graduating, too, and we had more or less decided that we would get together after graduation and really tie one on. After the morning graduation procession at Ohio Stadium, the Horseshoe, I returned to the house and really couldn't find anybody to celebrate with. Everybody just graduated and got the hell out of town. So that's what I did. My mother and brothers were there, and we just circled the wagons and got the hell out of Dodge and went home to Zanesville.

Well, here I was again, in a situation somewhat similar to high school graduation. After almost five years having changed majors three times and missing a couple quarters due to stress and being tired of it, it was over. I did what I came to do and had my degree. I was pretty sure that I wouldn't be able to get a teaching job due to the prejudicial attitude of public school superintendents at the time.

True, I had completed my student-teaching with a passing grade and supportive reports from my teacher-mentor at Whetstone. I thought that maybe in my hometown, anyway, where they knew me and my abilities and that I could perform beyond the norm of most visually impaired people, that I might have a chance of getting a job there.

Well, no such luck. I completed over one hundred applications and got two job interviews, one of them in Zanesville. They seemed to be preoccupied with how I would maintain discipline in the classroom. A genuine concern, I suppose, because of liabilities and such.

I put those worries aside for the time being and spent a wonderful summer of working at Camp Moores. Following the end of camp and after a trip to Canada fishing with three or four other guys, I got serious about trying to find a teaching job, but no soap.

My vocational rehabilitation counselor with the Bureau of Service to the Blind, Norman Young, a man that I admired highly, spoke with the local Goodwill about me and my interest in working.

I'm sure that Mr. Young put in a good word about my abilities and personality. From that, I got an interview with Rev. David Boldt, who consequently offered me a position at Zanesville Goodwill Industries as personnel director.

I was also to be in charge of rehabilitation programs run by Goodwill to try to get disabled people ready for work. I didn't know much about rehabilitation and the rest of the staff, including Reverend Boldt, didn't either. I muddled through, doing very little because I didn't know exactly what to do and was kind of left on my own to flounder around.

The best thing that happened to me during my time at Goodwill Industries was meeting my future wife, Vicki. Despite working full-time, I had also joined a local combo called the Jaquets. We were usually a weekend band, playing at local taverns, parties, or at service groups such as the Eagles, the Elks, and the Moose in a twenty-county area in Ohio and West Virginia.

While working a gig one night, I heard a lovely voice ask me if I knew the song "More." I did and performed the song for the owner of that lovely voice, who, I was told later, was the wife of another musician in the area. Back in the sixties, there were other music combos working in Zanesville, and the social climate was very active. Miss Vicki would come to town with her husband when he was playing another gig, and she would roam around from place to place in town to see who was playing where and what was going on.

We established an almost instantaneous relationship, she and I. She had two small children and was the only one in her family working steadily. Her husband, who was something of a ne'er-do-well, took dance jobs on the weekend but was otherwise unemployed and let her bring home the bacon, so to speak. Vicki was working as an unskilled laborer at a local factory and didn't really like the job. She had an infectious personality, and I thought she would be a good addition at Goodwill as a supervisor in one of the production floors.

I had her come in and talk with Mr. Boldt, who was duly smitten also, and since there was a vacancy at the time, she was hired. This was great for me since it not only gave me a good supervisor in the textile department, but provided me ready access to her. I learned quickly that she was very unhappy with her life and was ready and willing to get out of the unpleasant situation she was in with her (as I found out later) common-law husband.

This all happened in January of 1966 or thereabouts. In March, I went with a friend to the town where she was living, about fifty miles from Zanesville, and helped her move out one night while her husband was away on a music job.

I fell in love with Vicki very quickly, and apparently she felt the same way. That June we were married and honeymooned in New York City. I came home from the honeymoon to an instant family—two sons: Shon, six years old, and Jeffrey, two.

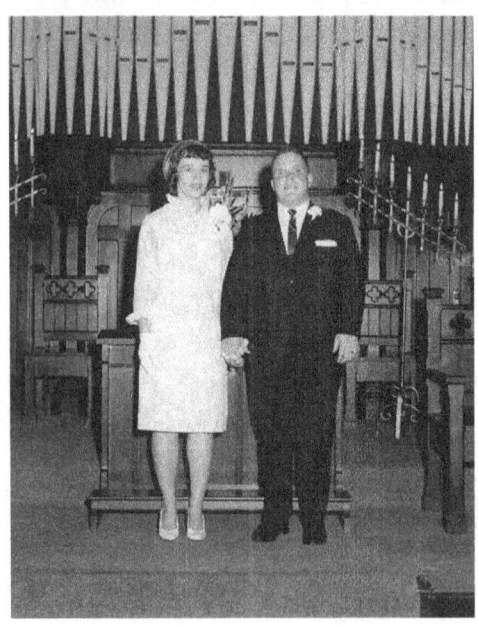

Jim and Vicki are married in Zanesville on June 3, 1966.

In terms of the challenges we would face as a blind husband and new father to her two children, Vicki and I talked about it some. But I guess I was in heat and thought I could work out just about anything.

I remember coming back from the honeymoon, I was very apprehensive about my overall ability to be an effective, loving father to two more or less young strangers, Vicki's children. I think, looking back, my experience working·as a summer camp counselor held me in good stead in that situation. We would meet the weekly campers on Sunday afternoon and live with them in a cabin of ten people until noon Saturday. That experience ultimately gave me a lot of confidence and skill in being able to read children and their emotions and learn how to make sound decisions based more on instinct than knowledge.

Vicki's feeling seemed to be that she didn't really consider me as disabled after having seen many of the skills and experiences I possessed, especially compared to what the children were used to in terms of their ne'er-do-well biological father.

I'm sure I made mistakes as a father, especially at first. Shon, being the oldest, probably had the most problems from my inexperience, but he turned out to be a dependable, skilled person and airplane mechanic who, unfortunately, later in life developed Parkinson's disease. Jeff, the second oldest, was diagnosed with ADD early on. But he overcame that very nicely, was in the navy for twenty years, and has been for decades a wonderful guy, provider, and father.

Steven and Mary, my children with Vicki, turned out to be successful and charming people. Mary has provided me with my only grandson, who, despite some inherited problems of his own, is becoming a wonderful young adult. So based on the above, I guess I muddled through as father and husband, and looking back, it was a great experience for me and, I hope, for the other members of the family.

My kids said it was tougher to have well-adjusted disabled father rather than a normal dad, because I had skills, especially in hearing, that prevented a lot of adolescent foolishness, especially in terms of sneaking out of the house at night. I quickly became attuned to squeaks and groans in the floorboards of the house and easily noted any sounds out of the ordinary. I'm sure that was frustrating to those bent on mischief.

I think we had a pretty regular life as lives go, despite my blindness. I was able to provide a good living for the family from my two jobs. We took vacations every year and visited with grandparents often, exposing the kids to different experiences and other relatives. They all, in turn, established their own families, living normal, happy existences.

Let me get back to the early family years. Vicki and I bought a house for the four of us and settled down, while I worked at Goodwill and took paying gigs as a weekend musician. And in December of 1966, Vicki gave birth to our son, Steven. We were now a family of five!

While working at Goodwill, I learned about a federal education program designed to develop highly trained, master's-degree-level vocational rehabilitation counselors. As I said, I didn't know much about rehabilitation. But now I wanted to learn.

The concept was interesting and viable, and the disabled population of the country sorely needed assistance in getting training, adjustment services, and jobs. The federal program was available at about sixty universities across the country. Included in the deal were free tuition, books and supplies, and a living stipend. I decided to apply for the program, and was accepted at the University of Tennessee in Knoxville, where I enrolled for fall semester, 1967.

Chapter 5: Tennessee and Wisconsin

In August of 1967, I resigned from Goodwill, and we all packed up and headed to Knoxville with Vicki driving the family car.

Kenny Weber and his wife drove our U-Haul containing all our earthly possessions down to Knoxville for us. They got to Knoxville a day before us and found the student housing assignment before we did. This was my first real taste of Southern hospitality as other students in the development pitched in and unloaded the truck before we even got there. They had the furniture placed, the bed set up, and cold beer in the refrigerator. Southern hospitality does exist, y'all!

I spent eighteen months at the University of Tennessee. I made it through the classes with Vicki's help, scored very well, and received a master's degree in 1969. I had my ups and downs as a student but got it done.

Two significant things happened while I was there. First, my father passed away from a heart attack in June of 1968.

I explained earlier that my father and I weren't really close. I never really felt like my dad accepted me as a handicapped person. I never felt comfortable around Leo and never was able to really talk to him. It seemed like anything I said to him was rejected or drew criticism. So when he died, I came home from Tennessee and went through the motions of the funeral, but I didn't really feel much of a sense of loss.

My mother's passing in 1982 was a different story. That was quite traumatic. She was such an integral influence, the primary source of strength in my life, that her passing left a big empty place in my heart. Mom's common sense, and the way she applied it to me in the challenges I faced, played a large part in making me into the person I am today. She gave me the feeling that I could do anything I wanted to do, and she reveled in my accomplishments almost as much as I did myself. All children should have mothers like Mary Sayre.

The second big event during my time in Tennessee was a happier one. I entered a talent show presented on a Knoxville TV station and won first prize—a $500 check, which was very handy at that point in my life, especially since we were living on a meager student stipend. In addition, part of the first prize was an audition with RCA recording company. The RCA people told me I had an excellent voice but gave me a polite brush-off, saying the material I wanted to sing wasn't commercial in their view. That's all right—at least we had the money, which gave us a nice Christmas that year.

Vicki was a great help to me in my schoolwork, assisting me with research and proofreading my papers. She was quite a bookworm. She also was there to read to me whenever I needed it. I must say the master's degree experience was much more enjoyable and less stressful than the bachelor's degree fiasco at OSU.

On weekends, Vicki and I and the three boys spent a lot of time camping and enjoying the nearby Smoky Mountains National Park, just forty miles or so away from Knoxville.

At UT, we often picnicked with friends of ours, Ralph and Joanne—Ralph was a member of my class at UT. We had a lot of fun with them, and they helped make the experience in Tennessee pleasant and acceptable. Vicki fit in with other wives in the Woodlawn student housing development and spent endless hours sharing with them over the building's washers and dryers.

There was a pool on the premises, and Shon, our oldest boy, learned to swim while we were there. One of the other students, being an enterprising young man and a licensed instructor, gave swimming lessons.

The living arrangement was probably the best housing I had lived in up to that time, certainly the best student housing that I have ever seen. It had the pool, tennis courts, the laundromat, a game room, and adequate storage.

Shon even had his bicycle there, but didn't ride it too much due to the extremely hilly terrain. It was fun going down, but hell coming up!

The last six months of our training was designed to be an internship, in which we would be assigned to an established rehabilitation office, either in the state program or in private facilities. I answered an ad in a rehab magazine one day and soon after received a call from Leonard Hoskins, director of Services to the Blind in the state of Wisconsin. We talked extensively two or three times, and he asked me to come to Milwaukee, where the central office was at that time, for a job interview. There was a vacancy, and he thought I would be a good fit for that position.

So we ended up traveling to Wisconsin for the requisite interviews with the dignitaries involved, and I was offered a position with the Wisconsin Bureau for Services to the Blind. This worked out great for us, as we needed the money from the job and I was also allowed to count it as my internship for UT. That left one other requirement to complete my studies, a master's thesis. Well, I muddled through that, too, after one of my UT classmates, Martha Walker, saved my bacon by retyping my thesis manuscript, which on initial presentation to the thesis coordinator was declared unacceptable. Martha was a highly intelligent and organized person and typed up my thesis almost overnight without a flaw. That version was accepted, and I was awarded my master's degree in 1969. I should say "we" were awarded my master's degree, Vicki and I.

Actually that's the way our marriage went for almost forty-eight years before Vicki, after a long and very courageous battle with cancer, passed away February 4, 2014. I've heard Vicki tell more than one person that we worked as a team together. When I needed help requiring vision, she provided it. Otherwise, most of the things around the house requiring repair or physical labor, I performed. When the task required vision and brawn, we worked together, usually harmoniously.

Vicki always claimed that she saw me on national television back in 1949 or '50 when I had been selected by ABC's *Kid and*

Company show as the saluted Kid of the Week, which showed my picture and told about my varied experiences.

Anyway, Vicki said at that time she knew that she was going to marry me. Farfetched or not, that was her claim. Fifteen or sixteen years later, that happened, and we were happily married for almost half a century.

We moved to Madison, Wisconsin, in September of 1968, where I assumed my responsibilities as a vocational rehabilitation counselor in the district office of the Bureau of Services for the Blind. I shared an office with a man named Richard Hunt, fifteen years my senior, and a native Badger. He ended up teaching me more about practical rehabilitation and the aspects of state-run agencies than any books I read in the master's program.

Dick was a unique person, very congenial, a navy vet from WWII who had lost most of his vision after developing multiple sclerosis. It didn't seem to hinder him much except that his speech was sometimes slurred. He was legally blind, but he got around well in terms of using public transportation, buses and the like, and walking. He did need a driver, however, when he went out into the community to meet his clients.

To understand his impact on me, you must understand that voc rehab involved a lot of bureaucratic procedures and requirements. In order to provide meaningful rehab services, you had to know how to navigate through the back streets of the system. When I got to Wisconsin, Dick had been a counselor for fifteen years and was really sharp about knowing how to bend the rules to get the best services for his clients. Luckily, he was a good-natured guy and didn't mind helping a nitwit from grad school learn the ropes.

Dick was also instrumental in introducing me to other members of the BSB throughout the state. Wisconsin BSB was a comparatively small organization, having about a dozen counselors covering the entire state.

The first week or two I worked in Wisconsin, Dick took me as a passenger on his forays into the hinterlands, so to speak. To get my feet wet, he allowed me to conduct initial interviews with new referrals and explain available services to the new visually impaired clients. In that way, I learned the services and the order in which they were to be provided.

It didn't hurt either that Dick and I shared a liking for beer and had many brewskis during our days. This not only helped me relax around him but deepened our camaraderie.

My area of responsibility was nine counties in southern Wisconsin, from Rock County (Beloit and Janesville) to the Mississippi River on the west. Not only did my area include several local breweries, but many cheese factories, as Wisconsin is the cheese capital of the country.

There was inexpensive beer and cheese and bratwurst in abundance, and of course, I liked them all. As a result, I gained quite a bit of weight in a short time and spent many years thereafter taking it off. I started by joining a running club for weight control at the local YMCA.

At this writing, I am sixty-six pounds lighter than I was at the zenith of my fat life in Wisconsin. What a chub!

Madison was a nice town to live in. It was pretty, had a lot of public parks and camping sites and many beautiful lakes, and the people were friendly for the most part. We decided, however, after a short time in our rented house, to buy a home in one of the many small towns surrounding the capital. We finally found a home we could afford in a town about fifteen miles from Madison called Stoughton.

Stoughton was known as the Norwegian capital of Wisconsin, and most of its inhabitants were of Norwegian blood. One of the main reasons we chose Stoughton was that it had a commuter bus going to Madison on a daily basis. This allowed me to travel back and forth to work as required and removed the necessity of Vicki driving me on a daily basis.

I've always excelled in traveling independently and was able to get around better than most, so the Madison commute was no problem. I've been able to travel alone to New York City, to Phoenix, to name a couple of places, and acclimated myself to new situations and living arrangements very quickly.

JIM SAYRE

Trip to New York City

Speaking of New York City, in 1968 I was chosen to be the representative from the Wisconsin Bureau of Service to the Visually Impaired to the annual convention of National Rehabilitation Associations, scheduled that year in the Big Apple. As low man on the bureau totem pole, I think I was selected because no one else wanted to go.

New York is intimidating for a lot of people, but especially so for blind people since we rely so much on our hearing. The level of noise was incredible, disorienting.

I took my white cane on the trip, because the theory behind the cane is to help others watch out for you, not vice versa. With the cane, I think it's other pedestrians' fault, not mine, if we run into each other. I mean, I can't see them! But the crush of people and the noise, too, makes it harder to stand out. The worst part of getting around New York was avoiding newspaper kiosks and especially entrances into subways—you could walk right into them and break your neck if you weren't paying attention.

I had been to New York once before, though, and had a grand time. Vicki and I honeymooned in the city and took in the *Tonight Show* back when Johnny Carson still had his show there. He even talked to us during a question-and-answer part of his monologue, asking us what the hell is the Y Bridge. An aide had collected questions and comments before Johnny came out, and I told him I was there on honeymoon from Zanesville, Ohio, home of the famous Y bridge.

Upon arrival in the city for my second visit, I was helped greatly by a friend who trained guide dogs and lived in Morristown, New Jersey. He picked me up at Kennedy airport and took me to my hotel, the Count Commodore at the corner of Lexington and Forty-Second Street. Then he was nice enough to walk with me on the route I'd need to take the next day to get from my hotel to the Waldorf Astoria, site of the conference. Just like my pal Joe Gormley did for me in the days before classes started at Ohio State, orienting me to the route I needed to know to get to classes on time.

One thing I noticed walking with the white cane is that most of the people who took notice of it and offered to help me were black. I think they felt that they saw me as a member of a different minority group who needed help.

But I met a lot of New Yorkers, white, black and Latin, who went out of their way to help me get around. One day I was walking back to the Count Commodore when a woman started talking to me. She insisted walking with me back to the hotel, then once we arrived, she said she was going to make sure I got to my room on the sixteenth floor. I wondered if she was going to roll me or if she was a street walker, but she just left me at my room and said it was nice to meet me. I think she was white.

Another episode of friendliness involved a hotel doorman with a thick Spanish accent when I was leaving to go back to Wisconsin. I asked him about getting to the airport, and he said there was a shuttle bus about a block away that would take me there. He decided to leave his post and take me to the shuttle location himself. So he picked up my suitcase, took me by the arm as we crossed the intersection, waited with me until the bus came, and then took off before I could tip him. I thought that was pretty neighborly of him.

Though I really didn't feel comfortable, I did go out one night by myself. The hotel was near a big railroad station—I think it was Grand Central station—and there was a bar in it. So I went in and had a few beers. Later, beer doing what it does, I eventually asked the bartender where the restroom was, and he said I had to go through the station to get to it. Well, that would be a problem, I thought. But some guy at the bar saw the white cane, intervened, and said he'd take me there, no problem. Nice guy. And the bar stayed open until 4:00 a.m.!

While Wisconsin was nice and the trip to New York was something else, Vicki and I never did stop missing Zanesville, the place this all started, and we wanted to get back there as soon as possible. We traveled back to Ohio each chance we got, but it was hard on Vicki since she was the only driver and the trip was some 550 miles one way. Quite a bit for her to handle, but she did it like a trooper, as they say.

Her ability to handle it was doubly impressive because when we got married, Vicki didn't know how to drive. We paid a private driving instructor through AAA, and after a few lessons, she obtained her driving license. It was doubly ironic because my job required a lot of travel, since we had to go from home to home or business to business to visit clients. If Vicki hadn't been able to drive me, I would have had to pay a driver out of my own pocket. She not only saved me a lot of money, but earned it by saving.

I'll wager that over my thirty-six years working as a counselor, Vicki drove me between seven hundred thousand and one million miles. Pretty good for someone who didn't learn to drive until she was twenty-six!

My family and I continued our enjoyment of the outdoors in the Badger State's many camping opportunities. We bought a pop-up camper and retired our long-suffering tent.

Try as she might, Vicki never got the hang of backing up the trailer. We'd get as close as possible to the campsite, then we'd muscle the damn trailer into position on its wheels and on my back—ouch!

One of our favorite places to camp was a state park in Wisconsin called Wyalusing, located on the bluffs overlooking the Mississippi River at the confluence with the Wisconsin River. A beautiful place.

We also visited the Apostle Islands in Lake Superior off the northern coast of Wisconsin, a place called Madeline Island. Also Washington Island in Lake Michigan off Green Bay. That was a real trip—it was real rough going out. The large ferryboat pitched and yawed and did everything but stand on its head! The kids were frightened, and so were we. We made it to the island and did our tour, expecting to return to the mainland later that day. As time went on, it became more evident that the weather was not improving and we'd be unable to return that night. We found a ramshackle cabin to rent for the night and settled down to wait it out. We were able to return to the mainland the next day once the weather calmed down.

Stoughton was something of a disappointment to us, so we decided to sell our house to move back to Madison, or closer to Madison. We couldn't really seem to break into the social circles in Stoughton. I consider Vicki and myself both friendly people, easy to meet and get along with. She usually was, I sometimes am. Anyway, we were unable to make close friends, even though I joined the junior Chamber of Commerce and did some volunteer work with that organization.

So we moved back to Madison, into a newly built townhouse apartment in the northeastern part of the city. I was able to use public transportation to get back and forth to my office, and it was okay. We soon found that apartment living isn't what it's cracked up to be. I suppose that depends a lot on the people who are around you in other apartments. Madison is a rather liberal city and even back then had a pronounced drug problem, which reared its ugly head in the apartment community. Several incidents there led us to believe it wasn't really a good place to raise children.

While living in the apartment, the director position of BSB came available. Mr. Hoskins, who had originally hired me in 1968, left for a job in Florida. I took the civil service test and sat for the interview, not really thinking that I had much of a chance and not caring one way or the other.

Lo and behold, I was selected to be the next director of Wisconsin BSB. Because I had no experience in administration per se, the program was set up to have me function as director but be a trainee also. There were steps outlined for me to complete, which when completed would ultimately give me the full reins of responsibility of the directorship.

Well, it didn't take me long to understand that I am not, was not, and will never be cut out to be an administrator. I wasn't really sharp in analyzing legislation from the state legislature and understanding the relationship between those legislative initiatives and my agency's operations. I missed several things that I should have seen in the governing of the bureau. My fellow staff members, people I was close to before taking the position, changed overnight and became fairly hostile. I didn't think I had changed, but I guess their perception of me, going from counselor to director, changed my stature in their minds. The only one who didn't change toward me was my friend and confidant, Richard Hunt.

Anyway, to make a long story short, the directorship of the bureau became one of my failures in life. After close to a year of blundering around and not pleasing anybody, including myself, I decided to forego the directorship and return to counseling. This had been made conditional on my taking the job, and the transition back to counseling was easy.

In the meantime, I found out that Vicki had become pregnant again on one of our numerous trips home to Zanesville. In January of 1975, Vicki presented me with our first and only daughter after three boys. And what a joy Mary is!

Chapter 6: Back to Zanesville for Good

I had been trying to find work back in Ohio since I concluded my graduate work in Tennessee. As we all know, the wheels of justice—and bureaucracy—turn slowly. A position in my hometown finally became vacant, and I applied for the job. Soon I was making arrangements to move from Madison back to Zanesville, Ohio, my heaven on earth.

When we learned that I was getting the job in Zanesville, we returned over Labor Day weekend, 1975, to look for housing. I contacted a childhood friend who was a realtor in the area, and he showed us several available properties. In essence, we only had about twenty-four hours to choose and ended up buying a home at 2124 Wilmer Street in Zanesville, where I live to this day.

Two friends of mine—Rusty and Terry, friends since my Camp Moores days—came to Madison to help us move. Terry drove our U-Haul truck, and Rusty drove our car, with the camper attached. Goodbye, Madison! Hello, Zanesville!

When we reached Zanesville the next day, family and friends were there to help us unload and set up. What a job! Setting up in our three-bedroom, one-bathroom house was a little difficult and very cozy.

Four kids, including three growing boys and an eight-month-old baby girl. Bunk beds became the bedroom furniture of the day. Mary slept in our room, while Shon was assigned the smallest bedroom, which he dubbed the closet. I am sure there are many walk-in closets today bigger than Shon's bedroom was then. But we made it work.

I began my job with the Ohio Rehabilitation Service Commission, Bureau of Services to the Blind, in October of 1975. I was assigned several counties to cover, similar in concept to the territory I'd had in Wisconsin. Vicki, as usual, drove me in my work from clients' homes to possible placement opportunities, agencies and businesses.

Our broad responsibility was to help newly blind and legally blind people adjust to blindness by teaching them coping and adjustment skills and to find jobs for those who qualified for work. For newly blind homemakers, we helped them learn how to function in their new circumstance.

Several definitions of vision impairment qualify people for services from the agency: severely visually impaired, legally blind, and totally blind. Most blind people have some vision; that's why there are different legal definitions of blindness.

Totally blind is self-explanatory: no vision at all. Blackness, no light perception, no LP. That's me, but there aren't very many of us.

Legally blind individuals have vision falling below the definition of 20/200 or less, with correction. A simple definition of 20/200 is that a legally blind person can see an object at twenty feet that a normally sighted person can see from two hundred feet. The definition expands when you put in the "or": or have a field restriction of twenty degrees or less. Most people have a field of vision much wider than that.

Severely visually impaired are people whose vision disability requires them to rely on magnifiers or something to improve their vision mechanically.

Now, of course, if I was in the position to counsel people on how to cope with blindness and do things for themselves, I had to be able to do it, too, right? On my initial visits, many clients may not have believed it was possible when I told them how I did everyday chores for myself and my family.

But I explained that blind people develop these skills out of necessity—and that they could too. Luckily, as I explained earlier, my mother was very permissive in terms of letting me try things, even when the tasks in question certainly would require vision in the minds of my sighted friends.

Blind people can do things that amaze sighted people by relying on personal experiences, training, and the ability to logically dismantle an activity step-by-step.

Vision, of course, is a critical sense. But it's just one of five that accompanies our senses of touch, hearing, smell, and taste. So when vision is removed from your life, you use your remaining senses. Even though they may not be as dependable and accurate as vision, with experience and a stubborn "try, try again" philosophy you can learn to do an amazing array of tasks.

Cleaning House

For instance, in cleaning house, a blind person learns to substitute a lack of vision by establishing patterns, by using your tactile senses, and even your sense of smell. In vacuuming the living room floor, for example, you learn to establish a pattern of moving the cleaner across the rug that works for you. You may start vacuuming along a particular wall, running the machine first along its base, going forward and backward. Then overlap your strokes as you move gradually away from the wall toward the center of the room. Do that slowly, always making sure to overlap your strokes, forward and back, until you reach the opposite wall and the entire surface of the rug has been covered.

To make sure the vacuum is working as it should, you may decide to sprinkle a small amount of cereal or crumbs to test it before starting out. But be sure to use something you can feel—that uses your tactile sense.

Dusting can be done using the same pattern approach as vacuuming. Here, however, you may want to begin by carefully touching the table or counter to verify whatever knickknacks or other objects may be there to avoid breaking them.

Cooking

Earlier I talked about my woodshop training at the blind school beginning in the fifth grade. Mr. Petzinger, the shop teacher, was totally blind but was amazing in his own right, being able to repair things around the house.

He went beyond woodshop to teach us that most tasks around the house can be accomplished without vision, but that you have to do it! Most of the methods are not foolproof but are dependable enough to be effective.

Take cooking hamburgers, for example. A blind person can cook a good burger by using several of his other senses. You can tell meat is cooking by smell, and you can also tell by the sound of the sizzle. To tell how done it is, you can time it, or you can carefully touch the patty with your fingers to tell whether the patty is getting solid or is still mushy, meaning it's got a way to go. So by computing cooking time, feeling the meat under your finger, and by the aroma, you can figure out if it's time to flip the burger. Then you use the same skills to determine when it's done.

And when choosing a frozen vegetable to serve at a meal, you start out by simply feeling the contents of a package. If the items are very small but rounded and not flat, you figure out that you've got a bag of peas. If the items are small about the same size but flatter, you've probably got corn. If there are several different shapes in the package, it's mixed vegetables. In that case, broccoli, cauliflower, and carrots are easier to distinguish by feel.

Of course, it pays to have an idea about what's in your freezer before you attempt to identify stuff. These skills are not foolproof, but they're dependable enough to rely on, knowing that you could be mistaken. If you're dealing with cans, sighted people can help you identify contents, then you can apply braille labels to keep track of what you have.

Nowadays, phones can help. Hold them up to a bag of mystery or a can of question, and an app will tell you what it is. That is, if you're young enough to learn how to use the damn thing!

Dressing Well

In terms of selecting clothes that match, there are tactile ways to mark clothes so that you know what color you have. These things are not always foolproof, but you play the percentages. Most of the time you come out ahead. And nowadays, phones have apps that can tell you the item's color, too.

Of course, you have to remember on your own what colors are said to go together so that you can put together an appealing, matching set of clothes. It also helps to choose neutral colors when buying socks, shirts or pair of shorts that more or less blend with everything else. Vicki was very helpful with helping me with my wardrobe by buying clothes that matched. Even though she's no longer here with me, her influence remains in terms of helping me buy things that go with each other.

But just like society in general, there are always some people who are more talented in these areas than others. It's a personal thing and often reflects the emphasis that people put on the task. Some sighted people dress well, I'm told, while others give it very little thought.

So accomplishing everyday household tasks without vision is a combination of using your tactile senses, smell, perception, common sense, and logic. I have been blessed with skills for all the above and count my blessings every day.

As Mr. Petzinger said, you have to do it!

Managing Money

Some things, frankly, require the help of an honest sighted person. When you get paper money, you have to rely on a sighted person to tell you the denomination of each bill before you can mark it to identify its worth.

For instance, if I ask the teller to give me ten $5 bills, before putting those bills away I must mark them in a tactile way to know what I'm dealing with when I pull one out of my wallet.

Each blind individual has his own way of marking bills. A five dollar bill in my wallet will have a small tear in its corner. A ten-dollar bill will have two small tears. I place twenty dollar bills in a secondary compartment of my wallet, away from ones, fives, and tens. I distinguish the more numerous one-dollar bills by not making any tears or notches. If I get a fifty-dollar bill, I fold it lengthways. For the rarer hundreds, I fold them end to end, doubling them over in other words. Nowadays, electronic bill identifiers tell you what domination bill you have when you slip it into the receptacle. These are useful, but when dealing with paper money, in most cases blind people still need help from a sighted person.

Coins are different, since they're different sizes, some have beveled edges, and they even sound differently when dropped on a hard surface. Pennies are like a small nickel. Nickels are bigger than dimes but smaller than a quarter. Dimes are about the same size as a penny, but they're distinguished by their beveled edges.

A quarter is a larger nickel with beveled edges, while fifty cent pieces are larger than a quarter with beveled edges. And they have a different tone when dropped on a hard surface.

Of course now, in the day of debit cards and charge cards, financial transactions are done automatically, removing the necessity of the kind of marking of paper money I just explained.

Now I pay most of my bills by phone, memorizing my credit card number, expiration date, and three-number security code and providing it to the prompts as requested. In this way, I pay all my bills.

However, these methods also depend on the mental ability of the person using them and the day may come when I am unable to accomplish these tasks.

Music on the Weekends

After a few months in Zanesville, Vicki and I soon found that my income from the job with BSB was not quite adequate to cover our expenses. What to do for extra money? Before leaving Zanesville for Knoxville, I had been a member of a musical combo. So I decided to go back to that as a side job to supplement my BSB income.

I began looking around for qualified musicians to help me form a group. I found a keyboard player, who after some practice together, was very adequate for my requirements. I also got in touch with an old friend from my earlier music days, a pretty lady named Connie, who played the drums very well and could sing.

Word of mouth is usually the advertisement for a group like ours, and it didn't take too long for the word to spread that were available—and good. We set out on a journey which would cover twenty years of weekend music in local clubs and other facilities. The money I earned from music was certainly important during my early years at BSB, especially. As time went on, salary increases at BSB lessened the income problem.

Work with our group—the three-person Crowdpleasers—not only supplemented our income, but gave me a needed outlet for my musical talent. I was lead singer with the group and also played the tenor saxophone and, to a lesser degree, the clarinet, instruments I first learned to play at the Ohio School for the Blind those many years ago.

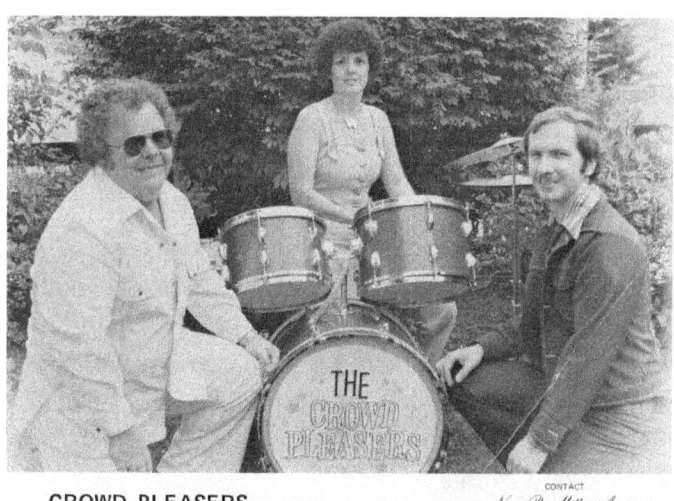

CROWD PLEASERS

CONTACT
Nina R. Miller Agency
P. O. Box 516
Beverly, Ohio 45715
(614) 984-2258

Jim with his bandmates in the Crowd Pleasers: Connie Touvell on drums and Mike Ward, keyboards.

I also worked on a project I had been considering for some time—an album of mostly music that I wrote. In my Camp Moores days, I had written a song or two generated by my love of the Muskingum River, which ran through the camp. While in Wisconsin, my homesickness for Zanesville led me to write several songs about my feelings for the area and my life growing up there. I couldn't afford this enterprise from my own pocketbook, so I decided to try to generate funds in other ways.

I was fairly well-known in the area, and when I started contacting different businesses in Zanesville to sell advertising for my project, I found people ready to help me out. We made placards and placed them throughout the community, advertising the businesses and people who had contributed to my project.

At that time, the city had an annual festival called the Zane Trace Commemoration, which celebrated the founding of Zanesville in 1797. The festival was held in June every year, and I hoped to have the album ready to sell by then. However, the pressing of the album was delayed, and I missed the festival and the income I hoped to earn there.

The project more or less flopped, and to this day I still have some vinyl records from the original one thousand that were pressed. I tell people that they make great Frisbees and targets for skeet shooting. But that project was less successful than I would have liked—to understate matters.

Upon my return to town, I reestablished friendships with Gary and Steve—two buddies from my early years in Zanesville. We all had a fondness for the Muskingum River, and we jointly bought a pontoon boat, which we docked at a local marina. We spent a lot of time on the boat and on the river, especially on weekends. Friday nights began a ritual where we would gather on the boat, have a few beers, and unwind from a week of labor.

Steve worked in industry, Gary in education, and I, of course, was with the BSB bureaucracy. We all needed to blow off steam.

One Friday night we were relaxing on the boat with some fireworks, illegal in Ohio, but that never stopped anybody. As usual, we were quaffing a few and firing off a few bottle rockets when the *Lorena*, Zanesville's riverboat, came chugging up the river on its usual well-attended dinner cruise.

I decided that the people on the cruise would be entertained by our fireworks and started sending bottle rockets in the approximate direction of the *Lorena*. Bottle rockets are designed to soar off into the air and, upon reaching their zenith, end with a loud, firecracker *boom*!

I fired several broadsides, and fortunately the dinner cruisers were highly amused. We received a healthy round of applause from them.

One night we decided to unmoor the pontoon and take it upriver to Ellis Dam, about seven miles north of the marina. We often cruised up to the dam, then turned around, sometimes killing the engine and just drifting back downstream with the current. This night was no exception. We killed the switch to turn off the engine and were happily floating downriver at about three miles an hour. But when we decided to restart the engine and head for shore, the engine wouldn't start, so we had to use the sole canoe paddle and a broom we had on board to try to reach the marina.

The broom wasn't long enough to reach the water without bending over, but I had broom duty and "rowed," bent over, to help us reach the shore safely. The next day I was so sore with a stiff back from the awkward rowing position that I could barely get out of bed. To make it even funnier, Gary, around noon the next day, found out you could also start the boat by pulling a cord near the switch!

The Crowdpleasers gained popularity, and we were busy every weekend, sometimes two and three nights. I remember one day we started out shortly after noon and ended up the next day about 3:00 a.m., having played three different engagements at three different venues. I had a good paycheck that weekend but ended up sleeping most of Sunday.

By this time, the three boys—Shon, Jeff, and Steve—had all graduated from high school and gone their separate ways. Shon completed training as an airplane mechanic and was employed by the Ohio National Guard working on their fleet of planes.

Jeffrey had entered the navy and subsequently was trained as a cook. He was referred to as an "airdale," doing cooking while on ship and procuring supplies when stationed on shore. Steven began college at Ohio University in Athens, but after a couple of quarters, he decided that academics was not his forte. He then entered the restaurant routine, beginning with a Zanesville franchise of a national pizza brand, then graduated to running restaurants. We were disappointed with his performance at OU, but college is not for everyone.

Ohio Bureau of Services to the Visually Impaired

Our life in Zanesville proceeded normally, and my work with BSB also entered a routine. Vicki and I continued in our workaday routine, me in my position as a counselor while Vicki provided me with reading service and transportation connected with the job.

In two different years, I was chosen as the BSVI statewide counselor of the year. This award was bestowed on the counselor who was considered exemplary by virtue of having the most successful closures, a closure being defined as helping a client find a job.

One year I was chosen as member of a "Dream Team," which meant that I excelled in a team-approach to rehabilitation and the successful placement of qualified clients.

While at the Bureau, I was chosen for the second time to receive the Charles W. Medick award as outstanding blind citizen of the year by the Blind Association of Central Ohio. The Medick Award honored me for "noteworthy achievement in his chosen vocation and for his example of courage, faith, and triumph over many obstacles."

I had earlier won the same award while working at Goodwill Industries in Zanesville after graduating from Ohio State. I was the first person to win the Medick Award twice, and I am proud of that fact.

Soon after learning of me winning the second time, my nephew Dick wrote to Archie Griffin, the Ohio State football legend and only two-time winner of the Heisman Trophy, asking him to send a congratulatory message to me. Archie very magnanimously sent me a picture signed, "From one two-time winner to another!" That was an unselfish, thoughtful gift which I cherish.

I helped clients find some interesting jobs during my time working at BSVI.

I had one client who had been a shop teacher in a local high school. Later, he lost most of his vision and became legally blind. After we helped him retrain as a furniture refinisher, he set up his own shop in a building he had built on his property. He did a great job in this craft and earned a good living for several years. Eventually he had to quit that job for other medical reasons, and after some further training, he became a vendor in our business enterprise program. He placed and serviced vending machines in his area, utilizing a driver to get him from one site to another. He held that job, making more money for several years before finally retiring altogether.

Another client was legally blind and also suffered from progressive bone deterioration. She not only had a great voice but an abundant knowledge of sex. So we placed her as a phone sex hostess. Not a real savory vocation, perhaps, but she made good money. We categorized her placement as "phone solicitation" to make the higher-ups happy.

What we did a lot of time was send people to our rehabilitation centers to learn, for example, how to cook as a blind person or how to study as a blind person, how to use recorders, take notes, whatever you needed to learn at that point.

We would decide what was needed, and then we'd help them get it. It wasn't up to me to do the teaching, we'd arrange and pay for it. But I'd sit with clients, talk to them to decide what was needed, and explain the process. That's where the counseling came in, sometimes just reassuring them that they could do it. The "I did it and you can could too" kind of thing. Like I explained earlier, with doing everyday chores.

A lot, frankly, was teaching them reality, that some of their thoughts and fears were bullshit. Like "You're not being realistic, and maybe it's because you're lazy. You're not really sincere." Sometimes I dished out hard love. But most people really wanted to do as much as they could. Some people were willing to take SSI, but most people wanted to make life more convenient for themselves, better versed at doing this or that. There were times that we had to close out cases because clients weren't functioning properly, they weren't following through, weren't cooperating.

When you first lose a faculty like your sight, you go through a mourning period. Just like when you lose someone who dies, but in this case, the object of your loss is your vision. You go through a lot of the same levels of adjustment that you do in mourning, like anger and denial. You feel bad, like you lost a close friend. Depression, a lot of depression. Depending on the person involved it can last a week, five months, a year. But our main reason to be was to try to help a blind person rehab to the point where they could be reemployed.

Often we would start out with mobility training, teaching clients how to use a white cane to get around. Instructors would show them how to use the cane, how to display the cane, how to detect things like curbs with the cane. Mobility training also includes a discussion about the laws of liability if you don't carry a cane. If I, as a blind man, go out without a cane and step out into the street on a green light, I could be held responsible for causing a wreck or for my own injuries.

That's a big reason I started carrying a cane later in life, once I found that out.

In more recent years, we began introducing clients to the talking computer and teach them how to type so that they can use it. Computers have opened up a lot of employment opportunities that we didn't have before. Talking computers and tablets, especially.

The influx of computers in our society, especially those with talking screen readers, which have become generally available and very sophisticated over the past several years, have opened up many jobs to the blind and visually impaired—jobs that were not available to them before.

Unemployment in the blind community is still very high, unfortunately. This new computer technology and equipment will, it seems likely, lessen these rates as its access spreads more widely to blind people. I placed blind people in education, a field closed to me upon my graduation to OSU, but now with the new technology the field is opening up even more to us.

Back in the day, there were jobs that blind people typically did, like caning chairs and making baskets out of wicker, tuning pianos, making brooms. Other blind people were organists in roller rinks, that kind of thing. Some sat on corners and sold pencils, sold newspapers. Many blind people were relegated to these tasks. In fact, the blind school had courses teaching some of these different activities.

We carried that a little further. We had a program called the business enterprise program that taught people like the old shop teacher how to operate vending facilities, candy stores, and cafeterias. They'd manage the place, sometimes with others. I had one blind client who ran a college cafeteria with sighted employees who would do the cooking. It was a big operation. They made a good living—some of them made five or six figures a year. That was a good program.

Others were doing similar things in state office buildings. In interstate rest areas, a lot of the vending machines are operated by blind people who came out of the business enterprise program. There was a law—I'm not sure it's still an active law—that gave the blind the first crack at operating vending facilities and food stands in government buildings.

Chapter 7: Travel, Retirement, and Tragedy

In 1998, I took a solo trip to England, where I met friends and other walkers in Oxford and set out on what was called euphemistically a "camel walk" from Oxford to Cambridge, a total of ninety miles, in six days. The walk was designed to raise funds for church-operated mission schools in Kenya to educate children of the Gabra tribe.

The camel was symbolic as the Gabra tribe was nomadic and they relied heavily on camels in those travels. A camel met us at different locations during our walk and served for photo ops. I supplied music in churches and for families we stayed with along the way, singing and playing the guitar. It was a very interesting and fulfilling journey for me, made possible for me by contacts with Willits Sawyer, my oldest friend on earth, my nursery school pal from the 1940s.

I had another interesting experience in 1998, a result of family ties. My mother was born Mary Glenn and grew up in Cambridge, Ohio, some thirty miles east of Zanesville. Her first cousin was John Glenn—yes, that John Glenn, first American to orbit the earth and later, US senator from Ohio. He had grown up in New Concord, a town in east Muskingum County not far from Cambridge, the county seat of neighboring Guernsey County.

The way the family births worked out, however, John was much closer in age to my oldest brother Bob, born Robert Glenn Sayre. Bob grew up with John, and they saw each other often during their childhoods, with Bob in Zanesville and John, known to the family as Bud, in New Concord. In fact, when John first ran for the Senate in 1964, Bob—a talented journalist and writer—took a sabbatical from his position as news bureau manager at Nationwide Insurance head-quarters in Columbus to work on the campaign. Bob wrote speeches and handled press duties until John had a fall and was too injured to continue his quest.

John and Bob maintained contact through the years and when John returned to space as the oldest astronaut ever, at seventy-seven, while simultaneously serving as US senator from Ohio, he sent Bob two tickets to watch the launch from Cape Kennedy. Bob, being the very generous person he'd always been, invited me to go with him to experience the launch.

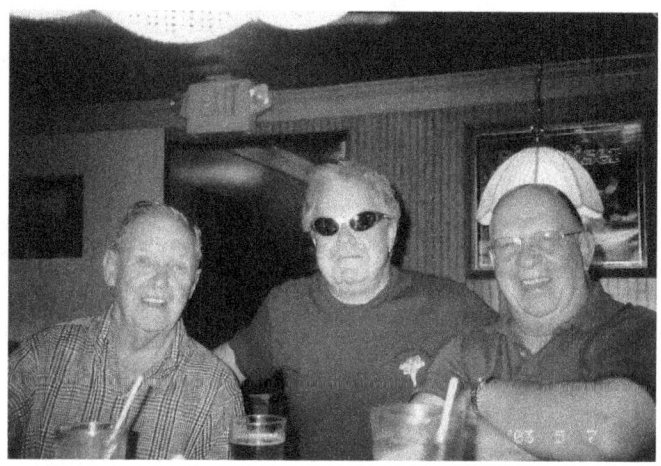

Jim with his brothers in 2003: Bob on the left, Ken on the right.

Vicki and I traveled to Central Florida about five days before the launch to visit with Bob and his wife, Sally, both then retired in Deltona. Vicki and nephew Bob, brother Bob's son and another Buckeye transplant in Florida, were unable to go into the visitors' section with us, but watched the launch with thousands of others from the surrounding area beaches.

Brother Bob and I were seated about three miles from the launch site, which was as close as any civilian observer was allowed. Even though I couldn't see the launch, I enjoyed it using my other senses—of course, hearing the roar of the rockets was unbelievable. I was unable to hear anyone or anything but the noise from the propulsion system for about a minute and a half, I'd say, until the space-ship achieved enough height to lessen the shock waves.

At launch, I could feel vibrations from liftoff in the ground and in a plate glass window in the building that we were standing just in front of. I felt the window moving back and forth under my hand as though someone was pushing on it from the inside—I was amazed it didn't crack! The glass must have been specially glazed to withstand extraordinary pressure.

I'm sure I didn't get the same impact as those who could see the smoke and fire, as well as hear the roar, but it was an unbelievable experience that I'll never forget.

I had a favorite aunt, Aunt Mary Sayre—now long gone—who was fond of saying that what I had accomplished over the years as a blind person was more noteworthy to her than the deeds of John Glenn. In my estimation, this was comparing apples to oranges, but we were both highly motivated and accomplished.

In 2001, Vicki learned that she had breast cancer. What a shock. How frightening to contemplate life without this wonderful partner. Vicki bravely underwent the recommended treatment and did accomplish remission. In 2003, our daughter Mary was married, and she being our last child to leave home, Vicki and I decided that it was time for retirement; we had things to do.

I retired from the Ohio Bureau of Service for the Visually Impaired in June of 2004. We had a great retirement celebration that included my family and many good friends. I entertained the guests during the dinner—always a ham!

Vicki and I decided to do some serious traveling after my retire-ment, but it wasn't long until other blind employees from the BSVI learned that Vicki, as an experienced driver and counselor assistant, was available and may be interested in further employment. Of course, this left me at home to do the bulk of the house cleaning, laundry, etc.—a complete reversal of our roles! There was, as they say, something wrong with that picture.

We did manage, however, to work into our busy schedules an Alaska cruise and a two-week trip to Hawaii. Of course, we were used to traveling since Vicki was from Maine and we loved to travel to that beautiful state to visit her relatives. She had an interesting family, and her parents had a comfortable cabin on Moosehead Lake, the largest lake in Maine. What's not to like?

We also traveled extensively in the United States, visiting relatives in Florida and other welcome destinations. After all, if you live in Ohio and you have relatives in Florida, you're supposed to visit them. Especially in the winter.

And we spent much time visiting our children, who, after following different paths, all gravitated back to the state of Ohio and lived within a two-and-a-half-hour drive at most from Zanesville.

I continued to work out five days a week or so at health clubs in the area and in my basement—and I still do. We've also had collection of dogs through the years which I have walked religiously, sometimes five miles a day. It has helped me retain a modicum of fitness, and Vicki even started working out with me in the late 1990s.

In 2010 I was included in Zanesville High School's Hall of Fame as the first blind person to graduate from ZHS and for my later accomplishments. People in the Hall had succeeded in their livelihoods and their communities, so it was a distinct honor for me to add my name to many other distinguished graduates.

Also in 2010, my dear Vicki's health was further impaired when, due to severe colitis, she underwent a colostomy, which was permanent. She spent forty-three days in a nursing facility following this major surgery, mostly flat on her back. Whether this was good or not remains to be seen, but she did deteriorate, and when she returned home, she and I spent many a day rehabilitating her atrophied muscles. We began by walking around the house, with me supporting her. Then we graduated to walking a block, then to other increased neighborhood forays. She was always a trouper and cooperated fully, ultimately becoming able enough to return to part-time work as a counselor's assistant and driver.

Unfortunately, I lost my lovely Vicki, who finally succumbed after some thirteen years fighting breast cancer. She left this earth February 4, 2014, with daughter Mary and me holding her in our arms, along with son Jeff's wife, Kathy. I lost the love of my life. I was left without Vicki.

Thus I embarked on one of the hardest journeys of my life. Not only having to do without Vicki's help, love, and support, but having to go on supporting our children, of which there were now only three. Stephen—Vicki's and my firstborn—had passed away due to kidney complications two years earlier, in 2012.

How do you make it through times like this? This was one of the hardest battles I've ever fought. Apparently I'm winning that battle, too, since I'm still here and doing comparatively well.

But I had some crucial help during the initial weeks and months following Vicki's passing from my brother Ken and his wife, Gretchen, who live a mile or so away. They had me over for dinner every night for months, helping to keep me together and fill the hole in my life. And Kenny would read my mail and give me rides if I needed one. Incidentally, Gretchen, my sister-in-law, is the same girl next door who helped me learn to ride a bike as a kid.

Until recent years, I continued to take annual canoe trips with friends from the Zanesville area. We would travel to Oil City, Pennsylvania, located in the northwest part of the state on the Allegheny River, and then go another eighty miles north to the Kinzua reservoir. There we'd begin a three-day trip down the river to Oil City. This annual happening went on for many years, and I was certainly happy to be part of the tradition while it lasted. Advancing age of the participants finally brought an end to the fun.

In April 2017, I left with seven other adolescent adult males on a ten-day sailing cruise of the Virgin Islands. This was a bucket-list activity and fulfilled all aspect of such an undertaking. We left from St. Thomas April 18 and toured St. John's, Tortola, and other islands in the area. People were so friendly and nice, and the place was so beautiful.

There was one tourist attraction in the area, supposedly an old pirate ship called the *Willie T.* The tradition there was to jump naked from the upper deck into the bay. After landing in the drink, you swim to a stairway and climb out, trying to hide everything, feeling very sheepish, and wishing you were better endowed. One of the guys on the cruise with me, Doug, jumped in before me to provide a voice target. I jumped and was rewarded with salt water up the nose, but knowing, too, that I may have been the first blind person to abandon ship in this manner.

My daughter Mary and I have continued the travel tradition established by Vicki and me. Mary and I twice have been to Ireland, Wales, and England, England being the land of our Sayre forefathers. She and I are planning additional trips to Europe, possibly to Italy.

Vicki and I had twice traveled to Iceland to visit our son Jeff and his family when Jeff was stationed there during his navy career. What an interesting place! Jeff and his family toured the island with us one year, even going to the Vestmannaeyjar Island, located a short distance from Iceland itself.

While we're discussing bucket lists and items on it, one of the items I've enjoyed twice now, once with Vicki before her passing and once since with Jeff and his wife, Kathy, is zip lining.

Zip lining for a blind person is not really that difficult. Of course, you don't get the visual effect, but a blind person still gets the feeling of motion, the wind in your ears and the excitement of stepping off a perfectly solid surface into space. I think the most exciting feature of the adventure—or the worst, depending on how you look at it—was the end, when you rappel from about a thirty-foot tower down to the ground. It takes quite a bit of talking to yourself to make the first step. However, zip lining isn't all that challenging since you're attached to the line and can't get lost.

I hit my eightieth birthday on Sept. 2, 2019, and had a party on a gorgeous late summer afternoon the following weekend out at the Headley Inn, an original stagecoach stop on old Route 40, the national road, just west of Zanesville.

I rented a large covered pavilion behind the inn, with trees above and a small creek beside us. Family came from Zanesville, the Columbus area, from Findlay up north in Ohio, and east from Maryland. They were joined by many friends from Zanesville— more than a few who've been close to me since high school—to fill up the place. We ate barbecue and beans, salad and bread, and birthday cake. Those who drink had beer available and those who don't, or thought it too early, had soda or water. Tales were told, old and new, men hugged me and women kissed me, and laughter rang out regularly.

I still feel good, still work out a few times a week. And I continue to meet every Friday for lunch with close friends, a tradition going on for many years now.

I don't know where my life will go from here, but I do know that I have had an interesting, loving existence. Like everyone else, I have bucket-list items that will never be filled in my lifetime. But this life has been fun, for the most part, interesting on the whole, and rewarding.

Acknowledgments

Growing up, all of us have had friends that are more than friends, or persons in our lives who have done more than just be friendly. I would like to acknowledge some of those people who have been important in my lifetime and thank them here.

To my mother, Mary Glenn Sayre: Your wisdom was far beyond your time. RIP.

My deceased wife, Vicki Roberts Sayre, you were my life for forty-eight years. RIP.

My oldest son, Shon Sayre, and his wife, Robin. My son Jeff Sayre and his wife, Kathy. My daughter, Mary Messick, and her spouse, Jason. My son, Steven, who passed at the age of forty-five. RIP, brother.

My brother Robert Sayre and my brother Kenneth Sayre. Thanks for your love and support and your wisdom when needed.

Nephews Robert and Richard Sayre, who have been friends more than relatives.

Karen Barnett, who has helped me fill a big hole left by my wife's passing. Love you, Karen.

Willits Sawyer, my longest living friend with whom I have done much mischief.

Joseph Gormley, judge and, before that, fraternity brother and friend throughout my life. The importance of that role cannot be told in words. RIP, brother.

Steven McGlade, Gary McGuire, Kenneth Weber—love you all.

In terms of writing this book, my nephew Richard was my invaluable partner. Working through personal grief and the pandemic, Dick listened to the tapes I sent him of my life's recollections, typed them into text, and then organized those words into the product you have just read.

In Zanesville, my friend Kay, on several occasions, read to me the latest versions that Dick had produced and provided several key edits to the story.

And my daughter, Mary, searched through homes and boxes to find the old photos that add flavor to my story.

I'm grateful to you all.

About the Author

Jim Sayre was born and raised in Zanesville, Ohio, a town that supported his dream to just be a normal kid despite his total blindness. Jim's determination to make that dream a reality led him to be the first blind graduate of Zanesville High in the 1950s. He later earned academic degrees from Ohio State University and the University of Tennessee. After some years outside Ohio, Jim and his wife, Vicki, and four children returned to his beloved Zanesville. From there, he built a career in state government while leading a musical combo on weekends in local entertainment venues.

Printed in the USA
CPSIA information can be obtained
at www.ICGtesting.com
LVHW040745131023
760664LV00002B/366